A Practical Guide to Using Qualitative Research with Randomized Controlled Trials

A Practical Guide to Using Qualitative Research with Randomized Controlled Trials

Alicia O'Cathain
Professor of Health Services Research
School of Health and Related Research (ScHARR)
University of Sheffield, Sheffield, UK

OXFORD
UNIVERSITY PRESS

OXFORD
UNIVERSITY PRESS

Great Clarendon Street, Oxford, OX2 6DP,
United Kingdom

Oxford University Press is a department of the University of Oxford.
It furthers the University's objective of excellence in research, scholarship,
and education by publishing worldwide. Oxford is a registered trade mark of
Oxford University Press in the UK and in certain other countries

First Edition published in 2018

Published in the United States of America by Oxford University Press
198 Madison Avenue, New York, NY 10016, United States of America

British Library Cataloguing in Publication Data

Data available

Library of Congress Control Number: 2017959068

ISBN 978-0-19-880208-2

Preface

Why the book is needed

It is by no means innovative to use qualitative research with randomized controlled trials (RCTs) in the field of health research. There are excellent examples in the research literature and also many insightful methodological reflections that have moved the field forward over recent years. In some research communities where researchers have long recognized the complexity of the interventions they are evaluating, the complexity of the environments in which RCTs are undertaken, or the complexity of communities or patient groups with whom health interventions are tested, this combination of two very different approaches to research is the norm. In other research communities, the addition of qualitative research to the world of RCTs may be viewed with suspicion and wariness. The book is mainly targeted at the first research community because even though it may be the norm to combine qualitative research and RCTs, there has been little practical guidance on how best to do this. The book may also be useful to the second research community, showing them why they might want to use qualitative research with RCTs and how they might go about doing this.

Although many researchers have combined qualitative research and RCTs, few have focused on integration of qualitative and quantitative data and findings in this context. Integration has been a neglected or invisible aspect of mixed methods research more widely and so it is not surprising to find that it is also invisible in this context. The book makes a unique contribution by filling this gap, detailing when and how integration can occur between qualitative research and RCTs.

The reach of the book

The book focuses on qualitative research, with its emphasis on subjectivity, flexibility, open data collection, depth, and context, and the RCT, with its emphasis on objectivity, standardization, measurement, and a key goal of bias reduction. The stark differences between the two methodologies make their combination a most interesting 'extreme case' of mixed methods research. Indeed the book sits within a framework of mixed methods research and more specifically mixed methods evaluation. Readers familiar with these areas will see similarities with these wider frameworks and also see how the extreme differences between qualitative research and RCTs provide some unique challenges.

The book focuses on combining qualitative research specifically with RCTs rather than the wider endeavour of experimental designs. Researchers engaging with pre-test post-test designs and controlled before and after studies in their evaluations, rather than RCTs, may find a lot within the book to guide their practice. The book focuses on RCTs because there is a research community of 'triallists' who live, sleep, and breath RCTs, and infrastructures such as clinical trials units to support the design and delivery of RCTs. The rules and regulations around RCTs present a particular challenge for qualitative research.

The book focuses on health research because the majority of RCTs are undertaken in this field. Health is a wide and varied field including health services research, public health, technology assessment, health promotion, nursing, rehabilitation, primary care, global health, and many more. The combination of qualitative research and RCTs is central to all of these sub-specialisms of applied health research and the book draws on examples from across a wide spectrum of them. Although the focus of the book is health, the combination of qualitative research and RCTs is also highly relevant to social and educational research.

The book is about how to use qualitative research when preparing for, or undertaking, an RCT. The focus is on a range of RCT designs including pilot and pragmatic RCTs. It does not explain how to do qualitative research or how to do RCTs; these issues are addressed in other excellent books. The focus of the book is how to undertake qualitative research in the specific context of RCTs.

Who should read the book

The book is written for researchers who undertake qualitative research before or during an RCT. Researchers often design and deliver qualitative research with RCTs without having studied how to do it because it tends not to be addressed in any detail at the graduate degree level (Masters or PhD). Researchers tend to learn through experience when they get their first job in this area. For this reason the book takes the reader through the process of a research study, from design to reporting, offering practical advice at each step.

The book may also be useful to researchers leading RCTs so they can plan well for the use of qualitative research with the RCT and understand the tasks and resources needed by their colleagues to best do their job. Researchers experienced at undertaking qualitative research with RCTs may also get something from the book because it brings together a diverse range of guidance and reflections in a single place. Researchers on funding panels, on editorial boards of journals, and who review grant applications and journal articles that combine qualitative research and RCTs may find the book helpful when making decisions about the methodological rigour of the research in front of them.

Finally, graduate students (Masters and PhD level) may undertake qualitative research before or during an RCT for their dissertation or thesis. The book offers practical guidance and a wide-reaching set of references within which to embed any empirical work.

The author's perspective

I will set out my beliefs and values here so readers can understand how these have shaped the book. Readers may hold different views and therefore disagree with some of the content of the book. I am happy with this—diversity of views can generate learning. My views are

- I think it is important to measure the effectiveness of interventions that attempt to improve health. RCTs reduce confounding and bias when measuring effectiveness. Because of this I support RCTs and do not attempt to challenge the 'RCT paradigm'. I do however recommend that researchers think about how they undertake RCTs and consider innovative changes that offer a better balance between the strengths and weaknesses of RCTs.
- I think that relying on RCTs (and accompanying economic modelling) as the only source of evidence of effectiveness is highly problematic. I believe that bringing other methods into play alongside RCTs, particularly qualitative research, can generate more useful evidence of effectiveness than RCTs alone.
- I want researchers to think carefully about the value of combining qualitative research with RCTs, to move beyond thinking about qualitative research as an addition to RCTs and think about the evaluation as a whole with the qualitative research and RCT as equally valued parts of it. The reality can be quite different, with qualitative research viewed as an add-on to the core of the evaluation—the RCT. My language in the book may sometimes portray this latter dynamic because this is the context in which I currently operate, but my goal is that researchers practice within an 'equally valued parts of an evaluation' paradigm.

Language

The term 'randomized controlled trial' is used throughout the book and abbreviated to RCT. In some research communities and countries it is called a 'randomized clinical trial'.

How to use the book

The book is written so that it is accessible to busy researchers and students who are likely to be reading it in conjunction with other books and methodological journal articles. It is short and easy to read with direction to further reading for those interested in delving deeper into the various topics covered.

Each chapter offers an overview of the material to be covered to allow readers to decide whether it is worthwhile reading the whole chapter. Key points are summarized at the end of each chapter to allow readers to digest the learning points quickly. Examples are described in most chapters within boxes to help readers who learn through examples.

Overview of the book

The book is divided into three parts:

- Part 1 Introducing qualitative research in the context of RCTs: overview of rationales, study designs and paradigms
- Part 2 Practical guidance for using qualitative research with RCTs
- Part 3 Engaging relevant stakeholders

Part 2 offers the practical guidance promised within title of the book. Each chapter focuses on key steps when undertaking qualitative research in the context of RCTs: writing a proposal, selecting research questions, collecting data, analysing data, integrating qualitative and quantitative components, and publishing. Part 1 is less about the practical side of doing this type of research—it sets the scene for the practical aspects. Part 3 is focused on the human beings we work closely with during our research and offers much practical advice to ensure these interactions are positive and fruitful.

As another way of making the book a practical guide, at the end of each chapter a small number of questions is listed to prompt readers to think about the projects they are designing or undertaking.

Acknowledgements

A heart-felt personal thanks to James, family, and friends, who always asked how the book was going. They made writing the book feel like an exciting process.

Professional thanks to ScHARR at the University of Sheffield UK for giving me study leave to write large parts of the book, Dr Vicki Plano Clark for encouraging me to write the book, the UK Medical Research Council for funding the methodological work that made the book possible, co-authors on the QUART study which spawned the book, colleagues who read and commented on chapters, and colleagues from around the world who do such wonderful research through combining qualitative methods and RCTs.

Contents

Abbreviations

GP	General practitioner
HIV	Human immunodeficiency virus
MRC	Medical Research Council
NHS	National Health Service
NIHR	National Institute for Health Research
PPI	Patient and public involvement
QUART	QUAlitative Research in Trials
QUARTER2	Qualitative Research with Trials: Excellent Reporting version 2
RCT	Randomized controlled trial
RE-AIM	Reach, Efficacy, Adoption, Implementation, and Maintenance
SMARTs	Sequential multiple assignment randomized trials
TB	Tuberculosis
UK	United Kingdom
USA	United States of America

Part 1

Introducing qualitative research with RCTs: overview of rationales, study designs, and paradigms

Chapter 1

Rationales for using qualitative research with RCTs

Overview

Read this chapter to learn about

- Definitions of qualitative research and randomized controlled trials (RCTs)
- Types of interventions where qualitative research is most relevant
- Reasons for using qualitative research with RCTs
- When not to use qualitative research with RCTs
- Relevance of qualitative research to different fields of health research

1.1 Introduction

It is common to hear researchers say they will undertake qualitative research to 'explain the results of the trial'. This chapter is about the wide range of reasons why it is important to use qualitative research with RCTs. Before addressing these, definitions of qualitative research and RCTs are given.

1.2 Definitions of qualitative research

There is no single accepted definition or set of beliefs about qualitative research but rather a variety of understandings held by different academic disciplines, research communities, and individual researchers. Some researchers may disagree with the definitions given below but they have been deliberately selected because of their relevance to researchers engaged with the production of an evidence base to improve health and health care.

While reflecting on the contribution of qualitative research to evidence-based medicine and health care, Barbour (2000) defines qualitative research as

- exploratory;
- describing, understanding and explaining phenomena;

- addressing what, why, and how questions;
- using a particular set of methods to generate data, e.g. semi-structured interviews, focus groups, observational fieldwork, document analysis;
- having an emphasis on context; and
- suitable for studying processes, how outcomes are achieved and mechanisms.

In the context of describing how qualitative research is used in the assessment of health technologies, Murphy and colleagues define qualitative research as involving 'the collection, analysis and interpretation of data that are not easily reduced to numbers. These data relate to the social world and the concepts and behaviours of people within it.' (Murphy et al., 1998, p. iii). These scholars identify key features of qualitative research as

- adopting perspectives of the people being studied
- concerned with description
- emphasizing context and holism
- emphasizing process
- flexible.

It is not always easy to categorize research as 'qualitative' or 'quantitative', and researchers take different stances on this. For example, some scholars use the term 'qualitative research' for surveys or for unstructured interviews where findings are reported as percentages (O'Cathain et al., 2014b). Neither of these would be defined as qualitative research in this book. The assumption in this book is that qualitative research involves both formal qualitative data collection (interviews, focus groups, observation, documents) and analysis (textual analysis, usually supported by quotes). This would include open questions from a survey only if the responses were rich in detail and an in-depth textual analysis undertaken. Qualitative research is distinguished from researchers' reflective reports on the problems that they encountered in running a feasibility study for an RCT, and from the use of methods that may draw on qualitative approaches but do not meet our definition. For example, research reporting the use of 'observation' and 'field notes' but showing no evidence of qualitative data collection or analysis in publications would not be classed as qualitative research in this book.

1.3 Definition of a randomized controlled trial

In the health field, a randomized controlled trial (RCT) is defined as

> An experiment in which two or more interventions, possibly including a control intervention or no intervention, are compared by being randomly allocated to participants. (http://community-archive.cochrane.org/sites/default/files/uploads/glossary.pdf)

The term 'randomized clinical trial' is sometimes used because historically RCTs have tested interventions in clinical settings. The term 'randomized controlled trial' is used in this book because it encompasses trials that test interventions designed to improve health in a range of settings including schools and communities as well as health care facilities.

1.4 **Types of interventions—it's not just about complex interventions**

RCTs are used to evaluate different types of interventions such as drugs, devices, and what are termed complex interventions. Complex interventions have several interacting components, numerous or difficult behaviours required by those delivering or receiving the intervention, different groups or organizational levels targeted by the intervention, numerous outcomes, and some flexibility or tailoring of the intervention (Craig et al., 2008). Examples of complex interventions include the introduction of lifestyle changes to reduce obesity, or the reorganization of health care delivery for stroke. A drug might be called a simple intervention in comparison with a complex intervention but Craig et al. (2008) point out that few interventions are truly simple. Indeed, the closer one looks at an intervention, the more complexity one is likely to identify.

There is an increasing understanding among scholars that many interventions evaluated in the health field are complex. Indeed, the growing understanding of the complexity of interventions has led to an increasing interest in, and use of, qualitative research at different phases of their development and evaluation. Although complex interventions are important to this book, and it is likely to be essential that qualitative research is used when evaluating complex interventions, qualitative research is relevant beyond complex interventions. A 'simple' intervention such as a drug may be used with a complex group of patients, for example methadone prescription for opiate addicts (Romo et al., 2009), or within complex environments, for example testing drugs in community settings in Africa to reduce sexually transmitted disease (Shagi et al., 2008). RCTs of these simple interventions can also benefit from qualitative research to engage with and understand complexities.

1.5 **Ten rationales for using qualitative research with RCTs**

The focus of this chapter is on the wide range of rationales for using qualitative research with RCTs. These rationales are not mutually exclusive but it may be useful to think about them in the following ten different ways.

1.5.1 To address a wider range of questions relevant to evidence generation

In the context of health research, RCTs are used to test whether new drugs, services, or technologies improve health. RCTs are considered to be the gold standard in the hierarchy of evidence of effectiveness. However, it appears that the question 'is it effective?' has become the gold standard question in an implicit research question hierarchy, when many other questions are important within evidence generation. Realist evaluation addresses the question 'effective for whom under what circumstances?' (Pawson and Tilley, 2004). Qualitative research can address questions about how interventions work (mechanisms of impact), how and why they are implemented in different ways, how context affects research and its results, and how to improve methods of measuring effectiveness.

1.5.2 To save time and money when generating evidence of effectiveness

It can take 5–20 years to develop an intervention, test it within a feasibility study, and evaluate it within an RCT. The process is likely to cost large amounts of money for a single intervention. It is important to develop as much learning as possible about the intervention and implications for other similar interventions to maximize the benefits from this size of investment. Investing in qualitative research in preparation for the RCT can help to optimize the intervention and give confidence that the full RCT is feasible. This can save money by reducing the probability of expensive RCTS of flawed interventions, or RCTs that fail to recruit. If the intervention is shown to be effective in the RCT, investing in qualitative research during the RCT can identify how effectiveness was achieved so that money is not wasted implementing a version of the intervention in routine practice that has little or no chance of attaining the size of effect found in the RCT.

1.5.3 To contribute to developing interventions with a good chance of being effective

Undertaking a large and expensive RCT of an intervention that is not well understood or has not been carefully developed may waste resources if the results are that an intervention was not effective because it was not feasible for delivery by health professionals or was not acceptable to patients. Questions about feasibility and acceptability of interventions can be addressed in preparation for an RCT. Qualitative research can be used to address these questions and contribute to the optimization of interventions and their implementation before they undergo expensive evaluation. Qualitative methods such as interviews and focus groups with those delivering interventions can explore what improvements are needed to interventions and how best to implement the new interventions in routine practice. Interviews and focus groups with those receiving interventions can explore improvements needed to the new intervention and how the intervention fits into the context of patients' lives and their management of their health condition. The example in Box 1.1 shows the impact that combining qualitative research and RCTs (and economic modelling) can have in the real world. The example illustrates the power of qualitative research when used as a first step to identify problems with existing services. This can lead to changes to services which are then evaluated positively in an RCT and finally implemented with success in routine care.

Box 1.1 An example of qualitative research as the first step in generating evidence of effectiveness

A research team in the UK carried out an RCT in Pakistan to compare outcomes of two ways of treating tuberculosis. The existing approach was by 'direct observation of treatment' by a health worker at a health centre daily for two months. The RCT compared the existing approach with a new approach which used more patient-friendly strategies of treatment supervision and patient support by community health volunteers or family members. The new approach was based on a qualitative study of 36 people attending a tuberculosis clinic. The abstract of the journal article reporting this qualitative research concluded that 'This study was performed to provide information to assist the researchers to design potential [tuberculosis] treatment delivery strategies, and has proved invaluable for this purpose.' (Khan et al., 2000, p. 247) The RCT showed that the new approach led to higher cure rates than the existing approach (Walley et al., 2001). This sequential mixed methods study, which also included a cost-effectiveness study, led to changes to government policy and public service guidelines and practices for tuberculosis control. The new approach was rolled out across Nepal and Pakistan from 2008, improving care for more than 300,000 people annually, reducing mortality rates and improving quality of life for people with tuberculosis.

Source: data from Khan, MA et al. Tuberculosis in Pakistan: socio-cultural constraints and opportunities in treatment. *Social Science and Medicine*, Volume 50 Issue 2, pp. 247–254. and Research Excellent Framework 2014, *Impact case study database*, available from http://impact.ref.ac.uk/CaseStudies/

1.5.4 To contribute to RCT viability and efficiency

It can be challenging to run RCTs. They can struggle to recruit sufficient participants, resulting in low statistical power, or there may be lengthy recruitment periods that require further funding. Qualitative research can help to improve the conduct of RCTs. For example, interviews with health professionals recruiting patients for RCTs and interviews with the patients approached for participation in RCTs can identify misunderstandings that lead to non-participation in the RCTs. Non-participant observation of recruitment practices can identify communication patterns that lead to these misunderstandings.

1.5.5 To improve the external validity of RCTs

The greatest criticism of RCTs is that they lack external validity because they recruit a narrow profile of the population that would be offered the intervention in routine practice. Pragmatic RCTs (see Chapter 4) overcome this problem by recruiting widely. However, some types of patients may choose not to participate in RCTs, even in pragmatic ones. Qualitative research can be undertaken with people who have chosen not to participate, or recruitment practices can be observed to identify any exclusionary behaviours in operation.

1.5.6 To explain the RCT results

In theory, RCTs producing null results are as valuable as those with positive results. However, in practice, null RCTs, which identify that interventions were not effective, can feel like a waste of time and money. In this situation, qualitative research can help to understand why the intervention was not effective and thus steer other researchers away from evaluating similar types of interventions and towards interventions that have a better chance of being effective (see example in Box 1.2). Alternatively, when RCTs produce positive results, qualitative research can identify the key aspects of interventions that contribute to producing an effect (mechanisms of impact).

1.5.7 To facilitate transfer of knowledge from RCTs to the real world

Policy makers, practitioners, and patients and the public want to apply evidence from RCTs to the real world. If an intervention was shown to be effective under experimental conditions, those wishing to implement these findings in routine practice want to know which aspects of the intervention are essential to effectiveness (mechanisms of impact) and understand the relevance of the context in which the intervention was tested to their own circumstances. For example, the control arm in an RCT may be the care that patients usually

Box 1.2 An example of qualitative research explaining the results of an RCT and guiding researchers to potentially more fruitful interventions

A cluster RCT of leaflets which summarized research evidence about decisions women make in their maternity care did not increase the proportion of women making informed choices (O'Cathain et al., 2002). Although the qualitative research undertaken alongside the RCT identified some problems with the leaflets, the main issue was that the culture of maternity care in the UK at that time was one of informed compliance rather than informed choice (Stapleton et al., 2002). That is, hospital systems and health professionals guided women to make choices favoured by health practitioners. The implications of this were that offering the research evidence in different formats such as through mobile phones would not address the fundamental problems of delivering informed choice in maternity care. The qualitative research offered guidance for future interventions to focus on the culture of maternity care to make it more open to informed choice.

Source: data from Stapleton, H., et al. Qualitative study of evidence based leaflets in maternity care. *British Medical Journal*, Volume 324, Issue 7338, p. 639. Copyright © 2002 British Medical Journal Publishing Group.

receive. The meaning of 'usual care' may differ by country and time. This has implications for the comparative effectiveness of the intervention in different countries and in different time periods. Qualitative research can help to understand mechanisms of impact and context and thereby guide understanding of the transferability of evidence of effectiveness.

1.5.8 To understand complexity

Complex interventions can be challenging and costly to evaluate because of their multifaceted nature and their dependence on social context. These complexities create methodological challenges for RCTs (Oakley et al., 2006) relating to difficulties in standardizing the design and delivery of the intervention, and understanding the characteristics of the local context in which the intervention is delivered (Craig et al., 2008). While an RCT may be the most rigorous way to evaluate the effectiveness of an intervention, qualitative research can help to understand the complexity of these interventions (Glenton et al., 2011) and the environments they are delivered within. This understanding may help policy makers, practitioners, and patients make decisions about how health care is delivered in routine practice.

1.5.9 To increase the relevance of evidence generation by listening to the voices of important stakeholders

In a methodological study of the use of qualitative research with RCTs, two public and patient representatives welcomed the use of qualitative research as a way of making heard the voices of two important groups when generating evidence: ordinary practitioners trying to help people to improve their health, and people with health problems (O'Cathain et al., 2014b). Qualitative research can help to identify the types of interventions needed, or feasibility issues with proposed interventions, so that interventions are relevant to those that will refer to, deliver or use them in the real world.

1.5.10 To improve generation of evidence of effectiveness

A qualitative interview study of 20 researchers in the UK who led the RCTs or qualitative research in mixed methods evaluations identified the following roles of qualitative research (O'Cathain et al., 2014a):

- problem solver: identifying problems at the feasibility phase to prevent them occurring at the full RCT phase,
- explainer: helping to explain the RCT results,
- translator: helping research users to understand the relevance of the RCT results to different contexts.

The interviewees also identified unintended roles of the qualitative research. These included:

- engager: engaging stakeholders who were important to delivering the RCT and thus ensuring the successful completion of the RCT,
- knowledge generator: offering insights into patient experience that had the potential to improve health and health care outside the context of the RCT.

An example of an unintended benefit is given in Box 1.3 where the qualitative research prevented further RCT participants using an intervention that early participants found confusing.

1.6 Thinking in terms of the value of qualitative research to generating evidence of effectiveness

A review of journal articles reporting the qualitative research undertaken with RCTs identified the potential value of the qualitative research to generating

Box 1.3 An example of an unintended benefit of qualitative research

Murtagh and colleagues (2007) undertook qualitative research to understand participants' experiences of the interventions in a three-armed RCT of a computerized decision support tool in patients with atrial fibrillation under consideration for anti-coagulation treatment. The researchers undertook a combination of non-participant observation and semi-structured interviews alongside the RCT. As a result of this the team discontinued one arm of the RCT because the intervention in that arm—a standard gamble values elicitation exercise—was causing confusion amongst the participants and was considered unlikely to produce valid data. The findings of the qualitative research raised methodological and ethical questions about the conduct of the RCT, 'ensuring felicity to the principle of non-maleficence, in parallel and complementary ways to data monitoring committees of RCTs' (p. 229).

Source: data from Murtagh, M.J., et al. Qualitative methods in a randomized controlled trial: the role of an integrated qualitative process evaluation in providing evidence to discontinue the intervention in one arm of a trial of a decision support tool. *Quality and Safety in Health Care*, Volume 16, pp. 224–229. Copyright © 2007 BMJ Publishing Group Ltd.

evidence of effectiveness (Table 1.1). *Potential* value rather than reported or actual value was considered because researchers rarely reported the actions that were taken in response to findings from the qualitative research. Some of these are described earlier in the chapter.

1.7 Six reasons for not using qualitative research with RCTs

Some researchers have raised concerns about using qualitative research with RCTs. These concerns may not play out in practice but are worth considering seriously as a way of attending to quality within this endeavour:

1.7.1 It is a fad—everyone seems to be doing it

In some countries it is common to undertake qualitative research with RCTs, in others it is unusual. Where it is common, some research funders may expect to see it in any grant proposal and researchers may include it simply to get the funding. This may lead to thoughtless use of qualitative research, the findings of which are then ignored during the research project. Qualitative research is likely to be far more useful in practice if it is undertaken with thought and because of its perceived value for a specific project.

1.7.2 It is an additional expense

Evaluations occur in the context of limited resources. Decisions need to be made about how to spend the limited research funds available. Qualitative research costs money and needs to deliver on its promise of making a valuable contribution to any evaluation, so that it is seen as a worthwhile investment. Oakley et al. (2006) argue that the additional costs of conducting process evaluations (which include qualitative research, see Chapter 2) are outweighed by greater explanatory power and an understanding of how well the intervention can be generalized. This is only likely to be the case if the qualitative research is high quality, and the findings from the qualitative research are listened to and acted upon. So although it is an additional short-term expense, under the right conditions it should be a worthwhile investment in the longer term.

1.7.3 It could damage the RCT

Some researchers are concerned that qualitative research may have an adverse effect on the RCT it is used with. For example, the qualitative research offers a therapeutic dose and thereby contaminates the experiment (O'Cathain et al., 2014a), or reduces recruitment to the RCT if additional commitments are required from RCT participants to join the qualitative research (Murtagh et al., 2007). These concerns only require consideration in the context of specific studies such as very small RCTs, when the qualitative research is intensive compared with the intervention, or when participants may be exceptionally sensitive to research burden.

1.7.4 Researchers already do this without using qualitative research

At a symposium on using qualitative research with RCTs at the Society for Clinical Trials annual conference in the USA in 2013 (SCT, 2013), the first question from the audience was why qualitative research is necessary when researchers undertaking RCTs do this work themselves without labelling it as qualitative research. That is, if recruitment is going badly within an RCT, researchers meet with recruiters to identify problems and implement solutions. The argument back from the researchers delivering the symposium was that it may not be possible to identify some key problems in this way because these problems are not understood by the recruiters themselves; non-participant observation or in-depth interviews might identify tacit behaviours in recruitment practices and offer further gains.

Table 1.1 Potential value of the qualitative research to the generation of evidence of effectiveness

Area of value	Potential value	Examples
Bias	Avoids measurement bias	Helps test face and content validity of instruments in the relevant patient group
Efficiency	Increases recruitment rate	Use of observation and interviews to identify problems with recruitment in a specific trial.
	Saves money	Stops attempts to undertake full trials of poor or unacceptable interventions, or use unacceptable trial designs Ensures full trials, which can be very expensive, are only undertaken on optimized interventions
Ethics	Makes trials sensitive to human beings	Recruitment and communication strategies can pay attention to health professionals and patients so that the experience is positive for them
	Improves informed consent	Challenges current assumptions about gold standard informed consent which values information over communication
Implementation	Facilitates replicability of intervention in the real world	Describes components of the intervention so that others can make use of the full intervention in the real world
	Facilitates transferability of findings in the real world	Identifies mechanism of impact or contextual issues important for success
Interpretation	Explains trial findings	Explains why trials were null. This may prevent another trial of a similar intervention Contextualizes results of successful interventions to support dissemination and transferability in the real world. Explains variation in outcomes
Relevance	Ensures interventions meet the needs of health professionals and patients	Identifies the value of the intervention to important stakeholders Ensures the intervention in contextually or culturally appropriate in different settings
Success	Makes a trial successful, feasible, viable	Engenders stakeholder support for the trial Makes a trial locally appropriate to cultural needs
Validity	Improves internal validity	Ensures right measures are used to measure right outcomes
	Improves external validity	Helps to broaden recruitment from hard to reach groups

Reproduced with permission from O'Cathain, A., Thomas, K.J., Drabble, S.J., et al. (2013) What can qualitative research do for randomised controlled trials? A systematic mapping review. *BMJ Open* 2013;3:e002889. doi: 10.1136/bmjopen-2013-002889. Copyright © 2013 BMJ Publishing Group Ltd.

1.7.5 It usually produces poor qualitative research

Some qualitative researchers will have no interest in using qualitative research with RCTs and may be concerned about the hijacking of their methodology to serve a quantitative master. They may view qualitative research undertaken in this context as shaped to fit the RCT paradigm, with an overemphasis on the utility of qualitative research, and a loss of the strengths of qualitative research. Researchers expressing such concerns are welcome voices because they help researchers who embrace the use of qualitative research with RCTs to reflect on their practice and move forward with thought rather than simply be swept along on the current wave of enthusiasm for this endeavour. It is important that researchers engaged with qualitative research and RCTs pay attention to the meaning of quality (see Chapter 13) and the production of high quality qualitative research.

1.7.6 RCTs are not appropriate in some contexts

Parry and Power (2016) argue that large-scale RCTs may not be the way forward for measuring effectiveness in the field of quality improvement in health care. They are concerned that not enough is done in an RCT to understand and influence the context into which an intervention is introduced. The scholars acknowledge the strength of qualitative research to understand context but suggest that alternative experimental methods to the RCT are required. Their argument, although this is not explicitly stated, is that the combination of qualitative research and RCT currently in use may not be enough to engage with the complex environments in which some interventions are used.

1.8 Different fields of health research

Qualitative research is used with RCTs in a wide range of health settings and disciplines of practice: palliative care, primary care, public health, health promotion, health technology assessment, health services research, nursing, medicine, and rehabilitation. Researchers in some health fields such as palliative care are highly engaged with using qualitative research and RCTs, offering reflections on methodological issues (Flemming et al., 2008; Higginson et al., 2013).

1.9 Key points

- Qualitative research can make a valuable contribution to developing and refining interventions, making the conduct of RCTs efficient, helping to explain the results of RCTs, and exploring context to facilitate transferability of effective interventions into the real world.

- Qualitative research is likely to be essential for use with RCTs of complex interventions and for RCTs of simpler interventions used with complex groups of patients or in complex environments.
- Qualitative research costs money and attention is needed to displaying the value of its use with RCTs.
- Not all researchers agree that it is beneficial to use qualitative research and RCTs.
- Qualitative research is used with RCTs in a wide range of fields and disciplines in health.

1.10 Questions to help you think about your study

- What is your rationale for undertaking qualitative research with an RCT?
- How will you know that it has been of value to the RCT or generation of evidence of effectiveness?

Further reading

Craig, P., Dieppe, P., Macintyre, S., Michie, S., Nazareth, I., Petticrew, M. (2008). Developing and evaluating complex interventions: the new Medical Research Council guidance. *BMJ*, **337**, a1655. doi: 10.1136/bmj.a1655.

Chapter 2

Frameworks, study designs, and guidance

Overview

Read this chapter to learn about

- Different ways of framing evaluations
- Frameworks and study designs for combining qualitative research and RCTs
- Different ways of framing the qualitative research used alongside an RCT (either within a 'process evaluation' or as an 'embedded qualitative study')
- The use of different labels to communicate the relationship between methods
- Available guidance for undertaking qualitative research with RCTs

2.1 Introduction

The use of frameworks and study designs can help researchers to plan their studies, communicate them to other researchers and stakeholders, and build up a methodological knowledge base to improve specific study designs. In this chapter different frameworks and designs are discussed in three contexts:

1. describing evaluations,
2. combining qualitative research and RCTs,
3. and describing the qualitative research when used alongside (or concurrently with) an RCT.

Researchers have started to produce guidance to help researchers to undertake qualitative research with RCTs. This guidance is briefly introduced here in relation to the frameworks described in the earlier parts of the chapter.

2.2 Framing the study as a 'mixed methods evaluation'

RCTs are often undertaken in conjunction with economic modelling and qualitative research. Researchers sometimes describe their whole study as 'a trial', 'a mixed methods randomized controlled trial', or a 'mixed methods intervention trial' (Creswell et al., 2009). That is, the economic evaluation and qualitative research are subsumed within the RCT. An alternative approach is to view the whole study as an intervention study (Sandelowski, 1996) or mixed methods evaluation consisting of an RCT, qualitative research, economic evaluation, and any other component. This last approach is recommended because it does not privilege one method within the whole evaluation, leaving other methods in the position of 'add-ons' to the main event. The significance of the language researchers use to describe their studies is discussed later in the chapter.

2.3 Frameworks and study designs for combining qualitative research and RCTs

There are five possible ways of framing the use of qualitative research with RCTs:

- a mixed methods study, drawing on mixed methods design typologies;
- an evaluation framework used for complex interventions;
- a temporal framework developed specifically for this approach;
- a 'process–outcome' framework where the design is concurrent use of a process evaluation to explore processes (with qualitative research undertaken within a wider process evaluation) and an RCT to measure outcomes;
- an 'aspects of a trial' framework built inductively from journal articles reporting the findings of qualitative research undertaken with RCTs.

2.3.1 Mixed methods framework

Using qualitative research with RCTs is mixed methods research, so it is important to consider this endeavour in the context of mixed methods designs (Creswell and Plano Clark, 2011). There are numerous typologies of mixed methods designs, none of which could be identified as the most relevant to this context. Creswell and Plano Clark's (2011) most recent typology is the simplest, broadest, and probably the most well known. They propose four major types of mixed methods designs: triangulation or concurrent triangulation, embedded, explanatory, and exploratory. All four of these could be used to describe different ways of using qualitative research with RCTs:

- **Triangulation**: qualitative and quantitative research are undertaken in the same timeframe with equal weight, e.g. qualitative research is undertaken alongside an RCT to explain the results of the RCT.
- **Embedded**: one data set provides a supporting role to a primary method, e.g. the RCT is the primary focus to determine effectiveness of an intervention and the qualitative research is undertaken to consider the acceptability of the intervention.
- **Explanatory**: qualitative research is undertaken after quantitative research to explain the results of the first method, e.g. after an RCT participants with different sizes of change in the primary outcome are interviewed to understand what facilitated improvement.
- **Exploratory**: qualitative research is undertaken before the quantitative research to facilitate the second method, e.g. non-participant observation of recruitment practices for an RCT prior to the full RCT is undertaken to identify ways of improving recruitment for the full RCT.

The timing of methods (sequential or concurrent) and the priority of methods (equal or dominant) distinguish the different design types. An example of a planned mixed methods evaluation is described in Box 2.1. Wiart et al. (2016) call their design a 'concurrent mixed methods study' but draw on triangulation a number of times within their published protocol.

2.3.2 Evaluation framework for complex interventions

In 2000 the UK Medical Research Council (MRC from now on) published a framework for the development and evaluation of complex interventions (Campbell et al., 2000), which was followed by further more detailed guidance (Campbell et al., 2007; Craig et al., 2008). The focus of the framework was evaluation more generally but it has been used extensively in the context of RCTs. The framework identified four phases of development, feasibility and piloting, evaluation, and implementation of a complex intervention, which researchers can move between iteratively. There is brief discussion of the contribution of qualitative research and these are articulated in Table 2.1.

2.3.3 The process–outcome evaluation framework

Process and outcome evaluations are undertaken concurrently. That is, a process evaluation is undertaken alongside a full RCT to help to explain the results of the RCT. A minority of process evaluations are undertaken after the RCT,

Box 2.1 An example of the use of a mixed methods design

Wiart and colleagues (2016) from Canada published a study protocol for a mixed methods evaluation of gait training for children with cerebral palsy. They describe it in the abstract as a 'concurrent mixed methods study comprised of a randomized controlled trial (RCT) and an interpretive descriptive qualitative design'. The RCT is a four-armed factorial RCT testing two different interventions used separately and together. The objectives of the concurrent qualitative component are to make clear the child and parent experiences of the interventions, the outcomes important to families, and the factors influencing participation in the RCT. The qualitative research is a semi-structured interview study of parents and their children who receive the interventions. Eighteen RCT participant child–parent dyads and nine parents who decline participation in the RCT will be interviewed to address the three objectives of the qualitative component. Families will be recruited from all three RCT recruitment sites because factors that affect RCT participation may vary between the regions and countries in which these health facilities are based. Interviews will take place at two time points: prior to patients getting the intervention and on completion of the intervention.

Source: data from Wiart, L., et al. (2016) Evaluation of the effectiveness of robotic gait training and gait-focused physical therapy programs for children and youth with cerebral palsy: a mixed methods RCT. *BMC Neurology*, Issue 16, p. 86. doi: 10.1186/ s12883-016-0582-7.

again to explain the results of the RCT. Process evaluations usually involve both quantitative and qualitative methods (Oakley et al., 2006). They are viewed as essential when evaluating complex interventions in order to provide insights about the mechanisms behind interventions, how interventions are implemented in practice and the context in which the intervention is being tested (Oakley et al., 2006; Glenton et al., 2011; Moore et al., 2015). In particular, process evaluations can distinguish between 'interventions that are inherently faulty (failure of intervention concept or theory) and those that are badly delivered (implementation failure)' (Oakley et al., 2006, p. 413). It has been argued that process evaluations are particularly useful in cluster or multisite trials to understand the context when the same intervention is delivered at different sites (Oakley et al., 2006), and when an intervention is trying to change the organization of health care delivery (Glenton et al., 2011).

Table 2.1 Qualitative research and RCTs within the MRC framework phases

Phase	RCT	Qualitative research
Development	Planned in the future	Develops intervention Identifies outcomes to be measured
Feasibility and piloting	Pilot RCT, or plans for full RCT in the future	Feasibility and acceptability of intervention, RCT procedures or outcome measures
Evaluation	Full RCT	Process evaluation or embedded qualitative study identifies how intervention is implemented in the RCT
Implementation	Intervention used in routine practice after the full RCT	Study of stakeholders influencing implementation in the real world

Reproduced with courtesy of the author.

The key functions of a process evaluation are to identify

- mechanisms of impact,
- implementation of the intervention,
- context (Moore et al., 2015).

Linnan and Steckler (2002) present seven key components of a process evaluation that can be addressed using either qualitative or quantitative research: context, reach, dose delivered, dose received, fidelity, implementation, and recruitment. Although it is possible to see how aspects of process evaluations such as reach, dose delivered and received, and certain features of recruitment or programme implementation can be assessed through quantitative methods such as checklists and surveys, others such as context and barriers or facilitators to successful implementation are more readily assessed through qualitative enquiry.

2.3.4 The temporal framework

A number of scholars who have reflected on the methodology of using qualitative research with RCTs draw on a temporal framework, which considers how qualitative research can be used 'before', 'during', or 'after' an RCT (Creswell et al., 2009; Lewin et al., 2009; Sandelowski, 1996). The RCT here is the full RCT (can also be called the main or definitive RCT) rather than a feasibility or pilot RCT.

- A *before-trial design* entails the collection and analysis of qualitative data before the full RCT, with the purpose of improving the subsequent RCT (Creswell et al., 2009), also called 'trialing the trial' (Sandelowski, 1996). The qualitative research can ensure that the full RCT evaluates an optimized intervention, recruits participants efficiently, and measures the right outcomes in a valid way. The focus of the qualitative research can be on the intervention, the trial conduct, or both. This sequential design is common, found in half of evaluations combining qualitative research and RCTs of complex organizational interventions (Lewin et al., 2009) and a quarter of more evaluations of a diverse set of interventions (O'Cathain et al., 2013).

- A *during-trial design* involves the collection of qualitative data during the full RCT to understand how the intervention is implemented in practice in order to explain the results of the RCT. A third of RCTs combined with qualitative research evaluating complex organizational interventions did this (Lewin et al., 2009). A process–outcome evaluation, described in Section 2.3.3, is another way of framing this during-trial design. Qualitative data is collected during the RCT and analysed prior to the RCT results being known (Oakley et al., 2006). Then the qualitative findings are used to explain the RCT results. An example of this is described in Box 1.2 in Chapter 1.
- An *after-trial design* involves collecting qualitative data after the RCT has ended to explore unusual results or the longer term implementation of an intervention. This design is not common, found in only an eighth of studies (Lewin et al., 2009). Sometimes, when qualitative research has not been undertaken during an RCT, researchers decide they want to do this after the RCT results are known because the RCT was null. An example of this is described in Box 6.2 in Chapter 6.

2.3.5 The 'Aspects of a Trial' Framework

A framework was devised based on the work qualitative research did for specific RCTs, as reported in published journal articles of the qualitative research findings (O'Cathain et al., 2013). Based on 296 articles published between 2008 and 2010, five aspects of a trial that qualitative research could inform were identified:

- the intervention,
- the trial design and conduct,
- the outcomes,
- the process and outcome measures used, and
- understanding of the health condition that the intervention addressed.

These aspects are explored in detail in Chapter 3. Most of the aspects identified in this framework were similar to issues identified by other scholars writing about this endeavour. The exception was the use of qualitative research to explore patients' experiences of the disease or behaviour addressed by the intervention under evaluation. This aspect was likely to have been a by-product of qualitative research which aimed to explore patients' experiences of the intervention. It may be problematic to set out with an aim of exploring patients' experiences of a health condition or behaviour using participants in an RCT because these are rarely representative of the population with that health condition. However, it may be an additional bonus for the mixed methods evaluation to understand something more about the health condition, especially if this has implications for the intervention under study.

2.4 Selecting a framework or study design

None of the frameworks or study designs described here are superior to others, although there may be expectations within specific research communities that guide the selection of a framework. For example, in the UK, the MRC framework for the development and evaluation of complex interventions is so well regarded that some funding bodies expect to see evaluations of complex interventions acknowledge this framework and follow the guidance. In the USA, a mixed methods framing might be more acceptable because a key funding body for health research—the National Institutes for Health—has produced best practice guidance for applications for mixed methods research (Creswell et al., 2011). Additionally, there is considerable overlap between the frameworks, and some can sit within another. For example, use of qualitative and quantitative research focused on processes and undertaken concurrently with an RCT can be framed as a process evaluation alongside an RCT or a during-trial combination in the temporal framework; this can be undertaken within either the feasibility or the evaluation phases of the MRC framework for developing and evaluating complex interventions. Researchers can draw on language for different frameworks. For example, Jack et al. (2015) use mixed methods design language to describe their process evaluation as a 'convergent parallel mixed methods research design'.

In Table 2.2 a range of studies using different combinations of qualitative research with RCTs are each described using the five framings described earlier. Qualitative research can be undertaken alone or with other quantitative methods such as surveys or analysis of routinely collected data. For simplicity only the qualitative research and RCT are described in Table 2.2.

2.5 Framing the qualitative research when undertaken alongside an RCT

Researchers use a range of ways to describe the qualitative research undertaken alongside an RCT:

- a process evaluation (Oakley et al., 2006),
- a mixed methods process evaluation (Sawtell et al., 2015),

Table 2.2 Framing the same studies in different ways

	Mixed methods	MRC Framework	Temporal	Process–outcome	Aspects of a trial
Qualitative research is undertaken to develop an intervention to be tested in an RCT	Sequential design Qual→RCT	Development phase	Before	Not applicable	Intervention
Qualitative research is undertaken in a feasibility study alongside a pilot RCT to explore the feasibility and acceptability of the intervention, and the feasibility of the full RCT	Concurrent design QUAL+RCT *or* Embedded design RCT(qual)	Feasibility/pilot phase	During	Process evaluation	Intervention Trial design, conduct and processes
Qualitative research is undertaken alongside a full RCT to explain the results of the RCT	Concurrent design QUAL+RCT *or* Embedded design RCT(qual)	Evaluation phase	During	Process evaluation	Intervention
Qualitative research is undertaken after an RCT to explore stakeholders' views of implementing the effective intervention	Sequential design RCT→qual	Implementation phase	After	Not applicable	Intervention

Reproduced with courtesy of the author.

- a qualitative process evaluation (Murtagh et al., 2007; Atkins et al., 2015),
- an embedded or nested qualitative study or process evaluation (Plano Clark et al., 2013; Masood et al., 2015; Lewin et al., 2009), or
- a qualitative component in a concurrent mixed methods study (Wiart et al., 2016).

Further description can relate to the approach taken to the qualitative research. For example, Wiart et al. (2016) use 'interpretive description' as their framework for the qualitative component, which focuses on subjective human experience.

Process evaluations usually include both qualitative and quantitative research (Oakley et al., 2006; Moore et al., 2015). When qualitative research alone is used, researchers may use terms such as 'qualitative process evaluation' or 'nested' or 'embedded' design. It may also be the case that the qualitative research is viewed as a separate endeavour from the RCT, with different teams, with any quantitative process data measured as part of the RCT. This occurred in the Healthlines study where a qualitative interview study alongside two RCTs was undertaken by one sub-team and the RCTs and quantitative process data by another sub-team (Thomas et al., 2014). The language used to describe the qualitative research in this study varied over time as the qualitative research team learnt more about this methodical approach. The qualitative study was labelled as a process evaluation in the application to funders because the qualitative sub-team had not understood the need to bring all process data together under this term. It was labelled as an embedded qualitative study in the published protocol (Thomas et al., 2014) because the qualitative research team felt that this more accurately reflected the study. Towards the end of the mixed methods evaluation the whole team discussed bringing together all the quantitative and qualitative process data as a formal process evaluation. In the final report to funders all process data was referred to as a process evaluation but the qualitative findings were reported in a separate chapter called 'process evaluation: embedded qualitative interview study' (Salisbury et al., 2017). The journal article reporting the qualitative research was called an embedded qualitative study because reviewers found descriptions of a wider process evaluation confusing when only the qualitative research was being reported (O'Cathain et al., 2016). This study was designed in 2008. If it were designed today it is likely that it would be conceptualized and labelled as a process evaluation alongside the RCTs, with both quantitative and qualitative process data.

2.6 **Language and status**

Drabble and O'Cathain (2015) reflect on whether the language used to describe qualitative research undertaken with RCTs can indicate different underlying assumptions about the perceived relative value of the qualitative research in relation to the RCT. The temporal framework privileges the RCT by describing other methods undertaken in relation to the RCT. Similarly the 'aspects of a trial' framework considers qualitative research in relation to the RCT. Both of these frameworks take an 'enhancement model view' (Popay and Williams, 1998) whereby researchers are interested in how qualitative research enhances the RCT, rather than how it makes a contribution to knowledge when an RCT is also used. The language of the process–outcome evaluation framework offers a more balanced relationship between the qualitative research and other methods in the study.

There has been some debate about the assumptions underlying the use of the term 'embedded'. Hesse-Biber (2012) suggests that 'embedded' implies a positivistic lens applied to the qualitative research, where it is given a secondary role as an 'add-on' to the more important and valued RCT. She argues that this limits the ability of the qualitative research to inform the RCT other than in terms of validating or confirming the dominant quantitative results. In contrast, Plano Clark et al. (2013) discuss varied understandings of the term 'embedded' and how it can be used to mean a high level of integration between methods, a description of a design where methods have unequal priority because of existence of primary and secondary research questions, or where the dominant method shapes the secondary method so that analysis and interpretation is limited. Plano Clark et al. (2013) then describe how using an embedded design resulted in a strong qualitative analysis and interpretation, that is maintained the strengths of qualitative research when used in an embedded design. In further contrast, the term 'embedded' has been used to describe mixed methods evaluations as RCTs embedded in qualitative research (Donovan et al., 2002; Hoddinott et al., 2010), signifying the way in which qualitative research has shaped specific RCTs. Adopting this different perspective allowed the researchers to take a dynamic approach to qualitative data collection, with feedback loops to the feasibility RCT (Donovan et al., 2002), and to step outside the bounds of the single question of effectiveness to consider contextual differences between clusters in a cluster RCT (Hoddinott et al., 2010).

There is no doubt that the current dominant approach to using qualitative research with RCTs is an enhancement model. This does not have to result in a loss of the strengths of qualitative research, and there are alternatives to this model, as discussed earlier. As this field progresses, a move to viewing the qualitative research and RCT as equally important components of a mixed methods evaluation may affect the language used. It is also the case that researchers may become more confident in using language that best describes a variety of approaches that can be taken. An example of this is Hoddinott et al. (2010) in Box 4.3 in Chapter 4, who use the term 'prospective mixed method embedded case studies' to describe how they assessed the effectiveness of an intervention to improve breastfeeding rates.

2.7 Guidance

Researchers have produced guidance for different approaches to combining qualitative research and RCTs. Future chapters in this book draw on this guidance, particularly Chapter 4. Readers are likely to benefit from reading the guidance in addition to this book:

- process evaluation (Moore et al., 2015),
- designing process evaluations of cluster RCTs (Grant et al., 2013),
- qualitative research in feasibility studies for RCTs (O'Cathain et al., 2015),
- writing mixed methods applications to National Institutes of Health in the USA (Creswell et al., 2011),
- multiple methods and RCTs in educational and social interventions (Grissmer, 2016).

2.8 Key points

- There are five frameworks researchers can draw on: mixed methods, evaluation of complex interventions, process–outcome, temporal, and aspects of a RCT.
- No framework is better than another but some are more popular in specific research communities.
- Qualitative research can be described as occurring within a process evaluation alongside an RCT or embedded or nested within an RCT.
- The language used can communicate status of methods, especially given a stance of qualitative research enhancing an RCT rather than both contributing together to evidence generation within a mixed methods evaluation.
- Guidance exists for using qualitative research and RCTs and is recommended reading.

2.9 **Questions to help you think about your study**

- How do you want to describe your study and why?
- How do you want to describe your qualitative research in relation to the RCT and why?

Further reading

Curry, L., Nunez-Smith, M. (2015). *Mixed Methods in Health Sciences Research: A Practical Primer*. Sage Publications.

Moore, G., Audrey, S., Barker, M., Bond, L., Bonell, C., Cooper, C., Hardeman, W., Moore, L., O'Cathain, A., Tannaze, T., Wight, D., Baird, J. (2015). Process evaluation of complex interventions. Medical Research Council guidance. *BMJ*, **350**, h1258.

Chapter 3

How qualitative research can contribute to generating evidence of effectiveness

Overview

Read this chapter to learn about the contributions qualitative research can make to understanding

- The intervention tested in an RCT
- The RCT processes such as recruitment
- Outcomes of an RCT
- Outcome measures within an RCT

3.1 Introduction

Chapter 1 described the rationales researchers have for using qualitative research with RCTs, such as improving the intervention, explaining how effectiveness was achieved or not, and facilitating knowledge transfer into routine practice. In this chapter, the focus is on drilling down to more specific contributions. These are related to the objectives or research questions of the qualitative research (see Chapter 6) and can also be emergent (that is, unplanned) contributions.

3.2 Four things to consider about the contribution of the qualitative research

1. There are different ways of phrasing the same contribution of the qualitative research.
2. The contribution must be considered in conjunction with the rationale for undertaking the qualitative research (see Chapter 1).
3. Some contributions are planned and others may emerge during the RCT.
4. Multiple contributions can occur in a single study.

For example, in a qualitative interview study, researchers may have the objectives to explore the feasibility and acceptability of the intervention. They could also phrase this as exploring how the intervention is implemented in practice. If researchers are undertaking a feasibility study for an RCT, the rationale for exploring the feasibility and acceptability of the intervention would be to improve the intervention content and delivery. If researchers are undertaking qualitative research alongside a full RCT, the rationale for exploring feasibility and acceptability would be to explain the results of the RCT. In this latter scenario, the qualitative research may also identify ways of improving the intervention. That is, the contribution of improving the intervention is a primary objective in the first scenario and emergent in the second scenario. Further, researchers may also explore aspects of recruitment for the RCT within the same interview study so that a number of issues are being explored within the same study.

3.3 Framing the contributions

The contribution of qualitative research to generating evidence of effectiveness can be displayed using one of the frameworks described in Chapter 2. The MRC framework for the development and evaluation of complex interventions (Craig et al., 2008), and the temporal framework of before, during, and after the full RCT (Creswell et al., 2009; Lewin et al., 2009; Sandelowski, 1996), are excellent candidates for this purpose. The 'aspects of a RCT' framework (O'Cathain et al., 2013) is used to frame the contribution of qualitative research in this chapter because it is based on research published in journal articles and identifies key issues researchers have found in practice and wish to communicate to others. Attention is drawn to the timing of the qualitative research in relation to the full RCT within each contribution, and the chapter draws on reflections of a range of scholars (Drabble et al., 2014; Creswell et al., 2009; Flemming et al., 2008; Grissmer, 2016; O'Cathain et al., 2013; O'Cathain et al., 2015).

3.4 The intervention tested in the RCT

3.4.1 Developing the intervention

Qualitative research can be used to develop a new intervention or service that researchers intend to evaluate with an RCT. For example, in Box 1.2 in Chapter 1, patients and practitioners were interviewed about an existing service for treating tuberculosis. This qualitative research identified problems with the service and a new service was developed that paid more attention to convenience for patients, that is improved the acceptability of treatment for tuberculosis. Qualitative research can also be used to understand practitioner and patient views of the content of an intervention as it is being developed, and assess early prototypes. This work best takes place in the development phase of the MRC framework and at the before-trial phase of the temporal framework.

3.4.2 Improving the intervention

Interventions are never perfect, and once developed significant problems can be uncovered as they are used by different people in different environments. Qualitative research can help to identify improvements to the intervention at all phases of the MRC and temporal frameworks. It is best if this work is undertaken at the feasibility/before-trials phase so that the intervention is optimized for testing in the full RCT. Even if considerable work is undertaken to identify and fix problems with an intervention prior to the full RCT, it is still likely that further problems are identified at the evaluation phase or during-trial phase. If significant problems are found during the full RCT, this may explain why the intervention was shown not to be effective within the RCT. If some problems with the intervention are identified, and the RCT shows the intervention is effective, then this may offer guidance to both researchers developing similar interventions and practitioners who will use the intervention in routine practice.

3.4.3 Describing the intervention

Qualitative research can be used to explore the extent to which the intervention delivered is the same as that articulated by the developers. Practitioners may have to adapt delivery to make it feasible or acceptable to them or their patients. They may add components to the intervention, and these components need to be documented as part of the intervention so that if the RCT shows the intervention to be effective it can be replicated in routine practice. It is best if this work is undertaken at the feasibility/before-trial phase but additional components may only occur during the full RCT as a wider group of practitioners and patients use the intervention. Practitioners may also not deliver key aspects of the intervention and this is relevant to the 'fidelity' and 'implementation' contributions of qualitative research described later.

3.4.4 Understanding how the intervention works: mechanisms of impact

The intervention may be based on a theory, with a logic model showing the causal pathways (see Chapter 6). The logic model is a diagram showing how different aspects of the intervention deliver the primary outcome via

Box 3.1 An example of qualitative research identifying a mechanism of impact

O'Cathain and colleagues (2016) undertook a qualitative interview study of staff and patients experiencing a new telehealth intervention in two linked RCTs for people with depression and people with risk factors for cardiovascular disease. The aim of the qualitative research was to explore the feasibility and acceptability of the intervention. A key finding was the importance of having motivated and enthusiastic staff delivering the intervention. This helped patients to engage with the intervention, stay engaged with the intervention, and take actions to improve their health because patients felt that someone cared about them. This issue was identified from interviews with 24 patients who received the intervention, some of whom had dropped out of the intervention or did not take actions because they felt some staff delivering the intervention were following prompts on a computer rather than thinking about individual patients' needs.

Source: data from O'Cathain, A., et al. (2016) Being human: a qualitative interview study exploring why a telehealth intervention for management of chronic conditions had a modest effect. *Journal of Medical Internet Research*, Volume 18, Issue 6, p. e163. doi: 10.2196/jmir.5879. Copyright © 2016 Alicia O'Cathain et al.

processes and intermediate outcomes. Quantitative analysis of pilot RCT data or full RCT data can identify relationships between variables along these causal chains. Qualitative research can also contribute to understanding how the intervention delivers outcomes by identifying aspects of the intervention that practitioners and patients associate with impact. It is important to consider this contribution at the feasibility/before-trial phase but it is also usually highly relevant at the evaluation/during-trial phase. This contribution is identified as a key function of process evaluations (Moore et al., 2015). The example in Box 3.1 shows how qualitative research identified the importance of having motivated and enthusiastic staff delivering a telehealth intervention. This highlighted the need for future providers of this or a similar service to pay attention to who delivered the intervention as well as the technology within it.

3.4.5 Developing, refining, or challenging theory

The aim of a realist RCT is to develop a mid-range theory to understand what about an intervention works and in what contexts (see Box 5.3 in Chapter 5).

The qualitative research can contribute to this aim. Researchers will not set out to use qualitative research to challenge the underlying theory of an intervention but this may occur as qualitative research is used to focus on implementation, acceptability or feasibility of the intervention.

3.4.6 Understanding implementation of the intervention

As practitioners and patients use the intervention in practice they may adapt it to their context and needs. They may use it as planned or may add, remove or reduce some components of it. If the RCT is null, this may be due to underlying problems with the intervention (see Section 3.4.5) or problems with how it is implemented (Oakley et al. 2006). Implementation is a key function of a process evaluation (Moore et al., 2015) and is important to consider at both the feasibility/before-trial and evaluation/during-trial phases of a mixed methods evaluation.

3.4.7 Exploring the feasibility of the intervention

Practitioners delivering the intervention may struggle to deliver it in practice due to the burden of delivery or the context of having a heavy workload. Seeking practitioners' views of important characteristics of any new intervention at the development/before-trial phase can facilitate its feasibility in practice; seeking their views at the feasibility/before-trial phase can identify issues that were not foreseen at the development phase; seeking their views at the evaluation/during-trial phase can identify further feasibility issues as the intervention is implemented in more diverse settings. The feasibility of an intervention may also be relevant to patients if, for example, they have to use a technical device that they find not to be feasible in their everyday lives, although this is usually described as 'acceptability' of the intervention.

3.4.8 Exploring the acceptability of the intervention

Intervention users or practitioners may find the intervention acceptable (Box 3.2) or they may be unhappy with some aspects of the content or delivery of the intervention. Some issues can relate to the practicalities of using an intervention, such as not using a telehealth intervention for monitoring of health behaviours because it is not conveniently available on a mobile telephone. Understanding what people value about the intervention can help ensure these aspects of the intervention are maintained if the intervention is rolled out more widely, while problems with the intervention can be fixed to improve acceptability. Patients and practitioners may have concerns about the acceptability of

Box 3.2 An example of qualitative research exploring acceptability of an intervention

Song and colleagues (2009) evaluated an intervention to enhance communication about end-of-life care between African Americans with end-stage renal disease and their surrogate decision makers. Outcomes were measured using an RCT and processes were explored using a combination of surveys and semi-structured interviews alongside the RCT. Interviews with patients and their surrogates identified high levels of acceptability although some wanted a further follow up session as part of the intervention. The interviews also identified what people valued about the intervention. In particular interviewees described how the intervention allowed them to have important conversations about issues they had not thought to discuss and ask hard questions that needed to be asked.

Source: data from Song, M.K., et al. (2009). Randomized controlled trial of SPIRIT: an effective approach to preparing African-American dialysis patients and families for end of life. *Research in Nursing & Health*, Volume 32, Issue 3, pp. 260–273.

the intervention in principle rather than in practice, for example beliefs that it is not appropriate to monitor someone's actions using electronic surveillance.

3.4.9 Understanding fidelity, reach, and dose of the intervention

Linnen and Steckler (2002) identify key components of a process evaluation (see Chapter 2), including

- fidelity (the extent to which the intervention is delivered as planned),
- reach (the extent to which the expected range of users receive the intervention), and
- dose (the amount of intervention received in practice).

These issues will be measured using quantitative data from the process evaluation but qualitative research can also illuminate them. For example, interviews with staff delivering the intervention and patients receiving it identified problems with fidelity of the intervention in that continuity of care did not occur as planned (see Box 3.1). These issues can be explored at the feasibility/before-trial and evaluation/during-trial phases of mixed methods evaluations.

3.4.10 Identifying the value of the intervention

A new intervention may seem like a good idea to researchers. If practitioners have to spend time delivering it and heavy workload is a contextual issue, or patients have to make efforts to use it, it is helpful to understand the value each of these groups place on the intervention and its intended outcome, as well as the amount of work they are willing to do to achieve the benefit. This contribution is often delivered by public and patient involvement (PPI) in generating the research question (see Chapter 15). If qualitative research is used to explore the value of the intervention of the outcome then this is best undertaken before developing any intervention.

3.4.11 Identifying perceived benefits and harms of the intervention

Early in the development of the intervention, users can identify the perceived benefits, harms or unintended consequences of the intervention, as well as their priority of any benefits. These benefits, harms, and consequences can then be measured in the full RCT. This ensures that the breath of relevant outcomes is measured in the full RCT (see Section 3.6.1). Perceived benefits and harms can also be emergent findings when qualitative research is undertaken in later phases of the mixed methods evaluation.

3.4.12 Understanding the context in which the intervention is tested

Understanding context is one of the three functions of a process evaluation (Moore et al., 2015). Indeed Hawe et al. (2004) use the term 'process and context evaluation' rather than 'process evaluation'. Wells et al. (2012) explore the role of context in RCTs. They do not explicitly explore the contribution of qualitative research to understanding the role of context. Nonetheless, their reflections are highly relevant to this book. Through the use of multiple case studies of RCTs of complex interventions they identified that context is important to understanding the mechanisms of impact, and the transferability of findings from RCTs of complex interventions. For example, context may shape the content and delivery of the intervention, fidelity to the planned intervention, the scale of the health problem addressed by the intervention, and practitioners' enthusiasm for the intervention. These contextual issues may affect the quality of the RCT conduct (see Section 3.5) as well as the intervention. An example of qualitative research attending to context is given in Box 2.1 in Chapter 2, where the researchers were aware of different approaches to treatment in the three regions and countries recruiting patients for the RCT. For this reason they purposively sampled interviews for the qualitative research by region/country to understand the impact of context.

An important aspect of context is the comparator arm of 'usual care' in pragmatic RCTs (see Chapter 4). Yet usual care can vary by geography and over time. This is a key contextual issue that may affect the extent to which practitioners or patients wish to participate in the RCT, the effect size achieved, and the feasibility and acceptability of the intervention (for example, it may be much more challenging to deliver than usual care in the context in which the RCT is undertaken). Usual care can be assessed using questionnaires in the full RCT/during-trial phase, with the content of the questionnaire shaped by qualitative research undertaken at the feasibility/before-trial phase.

3.5 Conduct of the RCT

3.5.1 Identifying effective and efficient recruitment practices

A large proportion of pragmatic RCTs fail to recruit, or fail to recruit within the original funding period. Researchers may have to stop their RCTs or request more money to meet the required sample size. Qualitative research can be used to study recruitment practices at the feasibility/before-trial phase to improve them for the full RCT, or to study recruitment practices during a full RCT that is failing to recruit in order to turn around recruitment. An academic group at Bristol University in the UK has developed a qualitative research-dominant intervention to study and improve RCT recruitment: the Quintet Recruitment Intervention (Donovan et al., 2016). Researchers employ mixed methods, including qualitative analysis of audio recordings of recruitment sessions, and semi-structured interviews with recruiters and patients approached for recruitment to identify issues such as lack of equipoise, or language used in recruitment sessions or participant information sheets that cause misunderstandings. Researchers take a dynamic or phased approach, feeding back results to the RCT team and the recruiters so that changes can be made immediately to training, language used, etc., during the feasibility phase or full RCT.

3.5.2 Improving retention of RCT participants

Some RCT participants withdraw early from the intervention or the RCT. Qualitative research with people who stop engaging at the feasibility/before-trial phase may be able to identify problems that can be fixed, such as misunderstandings about the RCT. This can improve the internal validity of the RCT, particularly if there is the possibility of differential retention rates in different arms.

3.5.3 Maximizing diversity of participants

A key criticism of RCTs is lack of external validity. Even in the context of pragmatic RCTs some patient groups may be difficult to recruit, for example people from socially deprived communities or ethnic minority groups. The evidence base generated is then not relevant to important groups because outcomes may differ by patient characteristics. Qualitative interviews with members of these groups and recruiters, or non-participant observation of recruitment sessions, can be undertaken before the full RCT to explore why under recruitment occurs and develop strategies to address problems. This may only be required for specific RCTs if the evidence base for a particular group is poor. For example, evidence synthesis has been undertaken to identify successful strategies for recruitment of ethnic minority groups for mental health research (Waseed et al., 2015). However, even with these strategies in place, some RCTs may require qualitative research for specific RCTs to identify tacit practices in operation.

3.5.4 Understanding impact of an RCT on participants, practitioners, and researchers

Some RCTs can cause stress to participants in the RCT, staff recruiting for the RCT or delivering the intervention, or researchers conducting the RCT. The potential for this may be understood prior to the RCT, and qualitative research undertaken before the full RCT to identify the stressors and ways of alleviating them in the full RCT. It is also likely that this issue can emerge from data collection undertaken for other purposes. For example, in an RCT of different ways of managing Type I diabetes, interviews with clinicians recruiting patients and informing them about their randomization arm revealed considerable emotional stress attached to these tasks (Lawton et al., 2015). The recommendations of this study were to offer further training to staff in future RCTs to help them to explain randomization and to deal with patients' anger and disappointment at being allocated to the control arm.

Practitioners recruiting patients might also harbour concerns that approaching potential participants for an RCT will be unwelcome, particularly when patients are in difficult circumstances such as having recently been diagnosed with cancer, or having recently given birth to an infant with a life-threatening condition. Qualitative research with potential participants, or those who have been approached and agreed or not agreed to participate, can reveal people's feelings about being approached and help to develop more sensitive recruitment procedures or alleviate the concerns of practitioners about the acceptability of recruitment procedures for participants.

3.5.5 Undertaking an RCT that is acceptable

An RCT may not be acceptable in principle because practitioners or patients have concerns about aspects of the proposed RCT design in terms of randomization or a placebo arm, or the feasibility of undertaking an RCT in a particular environment. If there are strong concerns that randomization or a placebo arm are unacceptable, then qualitative research can be undertaken prior to seeking funding for the RCT to identify the exact nature and strength of concerns. If there are concerns about conducting an RCT then a feasibility study can test the acceptability of this. Issues may also arise about the acceptability of the RCT during the full RCT. For example, patients may cross from their original allocated RCT arm into a different arm, prompting researchers to explore why this occurred (Thorstensson et al., 2008). Beal et al., (2009) undertook qualitative research with participants of an RCT of a wellness intervention for women with fibromyalgia syndrome. They were particularly interested in how the controls experienced the RCT and the existence of an active ingredient in the control arm. Here, the issue was acceptability of the RCT design to the researchers rather than other stakeholders.

3.5.6 Improving ethical conduct

Qualitative research can be undertaken to explore concerns about therapeutic misconception where patients might conflate research with clinical care, or where there are concerns about complicated informed consent processes. This contribution can occur when planning an RCT, resulting in simpler informed consent processes to improve people's understanding of the RCT (Penn and Evans, 2009).

3.5.7 Adapting RCT procedures to fit local contexts

Some RCTs are undertaken in complex environments. An RCT may not be feasible unless its conduct takes this environment into consideration. Community-based participatory approaches have been used to involve key stakeholders within communities in the development of the RCT. For example, Balcazar et al. (2009) undertook a pragmatic RCT of health education classes for cardiovascular disease prevention in the USA. They undertook community-based participatory research, including three focus groups with community members, to communicate the intervention and RCT to the local community. This research highlighted how to improve the RCT conduct as well as the intervention for this community. It also improved the human aspects of RCTs by treating communities with respect by undertaking RCTs with them rather than on them.

3.6 Outcomes of the RCT

3.6.1 Selecting outcomes important to patients and practitioners

At the feasibility/before-trial phase, qualitative research can be undertaken with the patient group to understand the range of outcomes important to them so that these can be selected for measurement in the full RCT. Qualitative research undertaken with people experiencing the intervention, perhaps alongside a pilot RCT, may identify further perceived benefits of the intervention (see Section 3.4.11). Comparison of these perceived benefits with what is planned for measurement in the RCT could lead to reassessment of which outcome is the primary outcome, or the addition or removal of some secondary outcomes. Practitioners may also contribute to this because they may value some outcomes more than patients. This contribution of qualitative research can ensure that the RCT results have more relevance to key stakeholders such as patients and practitioners.

Rather than undertake qualitative research with specific RCTs, a related endeavour is the 'COMET' initiative, established to minimize bias in RCTs and facilitate evidence synthesis of the effectiveness of interventions. Keeley et al. (2016) discuss the value of COMET whereby qualitative research with stakeholders is used to identify a core set of outcomes to be measured in *any* RCT undertaken on a specific health problem. The authors discuss the value of using qualitative research prior to a consensus exercise to identify a core outcome set.

3.6.2 Understanding variation in outcomes

RCTs measure outcomes on average. Qualitative research can pay attention to individuals and the variation in outcomes achieved, addressing why some patients show improvement in the RCT and others do not improve and even deteriorate. Differences between clusters or between individuals in an RCT can be explored. The qualitative research is undertaken during the full RCT. For example, Hoddinott et al. (2010) undertook qualitative research in the seven intervention clusters of their RCT and the used this to explain why some clusters improved breastfeeding rates whereas they deteriorated in others. Sampling clusters and individuals is required where there are a large number of clusters or individuals in the RCT. If sampling is necessary, it is better to undertake the qualitative research after the full RCT when outcomes are known and these can be used to select clusters or individuals that have had good or poor outcomes in the RCT. There are not many examples of this contribution in the literature (O'Cathain et al., 2013) and it is one that deserves further use.

3.7 Measures in the RCT

3.7.1 Identifying the accuracy of proposed measures

Measures planned for use in the full RCT may have been developed for a different context or different patient group from those in the RCT. At the feasibility/before-trial phase, researchers may use qualitative research to explore the face validity of key process and outcome measures they plan to use in the full RCT (see Box 3.3).

3.7.2 Improving completion of outcome measures

Outcomes measures in RCTs are often measured through completion of questionnaires by mail. Missing data or non-return of questionnaires can damage the internal and external validity of the RCT. If outcome measurement completion problems are identified in the feasibility/before-trial phase, qualitative research with non-responders can help to identify problems which can be addressed in preparation for the full RCT. Nakash et al. (2008) identified this problem in the full RCT and undertook qualitative research to show that some non-respondents had not understood aspects of the RCT, leading to non-completion of RCT measures; the value of this qualitative research was for future RCTs.

Box 3.3 An example of using qualitative research in a feasibility study to explore the face validity of a key outcome measure

Farquhar and colleagues (2010) undertook a pilot RCT of a breathlessness intervention for chronic obstructive pulmonary disease in the UK. The aim of the qualitative research undertaken alongside the pilot RCT was to explore the feasibility of using an outcome measure for the main RCT. Longitudinal interviews were undertaken with 13 patients in the intervention arm on 51 occasions. Recordings were made of participants completing the outcome measure. The researchers rejected the use of the outcome measure for the full RCT trial due to its lack of validity for their patient group.

Source: data from Farquhar, M., et al. (2010). The experience of using the SEIQoL-DW with patients with advanced chronic obstructive pulmonary disease (COPD): issues of process and outcome. *Quality of Life Research*, Volume 19, Issue 5, pp. 619–629.

3.7.3 Developing outcome measures

At the feasibility/before-trial phase, researchers may identify a range of outcomes important to participants in the RCT (see Section 3.6.1). If validated measures do not exist for all the outcomes, they can be developed in preparation for the full RCT. The first step can involve qualitative research to identify the items for the instrument, followed by the use of qualitative research in cognitive testing of early versions of the instrument. Quantitative psychometric testing can then be undertaken on a large sample of patients. Researchers have published articles reporting how they developed an outcome measure using qualitative research before a RCT and quantitative psychometric testing using the data from the full RCT (Abetz et al., 2009). The value of this approach was that it reduced the time and cost of undertaking a separate psychometric study prior to the full RCT. The value of the qualitative research was twofold: increased credibility of the results of the RCT because it used a validated instrument; and a validated instrument for use in future RCTs. The risk was that the psychometric testing might have revealed fundamental problems with the instrument and reduced the credibility of the RCT results related to that outcome.

3.8 Understanding the health condition in the RCT

A by-product of qualitative research undertaken with RCTs is that while exploring acceptability of an intervention, participants offer insights about the health condition the intervention is addressing (O'Cathain et al. 2013). Researchers have to be cautious when writing up these insights because participants in an RCT may not be similar to the general patient group. However, it can be a useful contribution where there is little or no qualitative research about a health condition (Toye et al., 2016).

3.9 Key points

- Qualitative research can make a large number of contributions to generating evidence of effectiveness.
- The same contributions can be described in different ways, and contributions can be rationale-dependent, multiple, and unplanned.
- Contributions include understanding the intervention, the RCT conduct, the outcomes of the RCT or the measures used in the RCT.
- Reading the range of contributions described here can help researchers widen their understanding of the contributions qualitative research can make and maximize the value of using qualitative research with RCTs.

3.10 Questions to help you think about your study

- If you are planning your study, what contributions are priorities for your study?
- If you are analysing your study, what contributions are visible in your data? Which of these are most important to address in your publications and why?

Further reading

O'Cathain, A., Thomas, K.J., Drabble, S.J., Rudolph, A., Hewison, J. (2013). What can qualitative research do for randomised controlled trials? A systematic mapping review. *BMJ Open*, **3**:e002889. doi: 10.1136/bmjopen-2013-002889.

Chapter 4

Using qualitative research with different types of RCTs

Overview

Read this chapter to learn about using qualitative research with different types of RCTs

- Explanatory RCTs
- Pragmatic RCTs
- Feasibility, pilot or exploratory RCTs
- Cluster RCTs
- N of 1 trials
- Factorial RCTs

4.1 Introduction

When researchers write methodological reflections on the use of qualitative research with RCTs, their focus is usually on individually randomized two armed pragmatic full RCTs. However, qualitative research is used with a range of RCT types. The objectives, data collection, or analysis of the qualitative research may depend on the type of RCT. Ways of using qualitative research with different types of RCT are described briefly in this chapter. Where guidance is available, this is described along with any challenges specific to each type. The opportunity is taken here to offer more detail about feasibility and pilot RCTs than other RCT types because methodological reflections have tended to focus on full RCTs and many later chapters in this book detail the more common practice of using qualitative research alongside full RCTs.

4.2 Explanatory and pragmatic RCTs

Explanatory RCTs are tightly controlled experiments, usually with a placebo as a control, aiming to measure effectiveness of interventions under ideal circumstances (Torgerson and Torgerson, 2008). Pragmatic RCTs are an alternative which offer external and internal validity. Their aim is to generate evidence that is applicable to routine practice, measuring the effect on an outcome of most importance to participants, practitioners, and policy makers and comparing it with usual care rather than placebo (Torgerson and Torgerson, 2008). The explanatory/pragmatic distinction is a continuum rather than a dichotomy, with researchers taking a more explanatory or pragmatic 'attitude' to their RCTs (Treweek and Zwarenstein, 2009). Those taking a pragmatic attitude favour decisions which maximize the applicability of RCT results to routine practice. Scholars have recommended that more pragmatic RCTs are undertaken because of their higher utility in the real world (Treweek and Zwarenstein, 2009). Because explanatory and pragmatic RCTs are on a continuum, researchers may only explicitly identify their RCT as pragmatic when it is at the extreme of the spectrum.

4.2.1 Explanatory RCTs

Explanatory RCTs are commonly used to test the effectiveness of drugs rather than more complex interventions. In a review of journal articles published between 2008 and 2010 that reported qualitative research undertaken with RCTs, seven out of 104 identified the use of a placebo in the RCT control arm (O'Cathain et al. 2014b). That is, these seven were at the explanatory end of the explanatory/pragmatic spectrum. The qualitative research used with these explanatory RCTs explored

- the meaning of the placebo to patients,
- adherence to the intervention,
- trial conduct concerning participation in the RCT and ethics, and
- the outcomes measured.

4.2.2 Pragmatic RCTs

It is much more common to use qualitative research with pragmatic RCTs because more complex interventions than drugs are tested using this type of RCT in complex environments such as communities, primary care, and schools, with usual care as a control arm. In the review described in Section 4.2.1, 12 out of 104 journal articles specified that the RCT was pragmatic, indicating that the labels explanatory and pragmatic are not necessarily used by researchers to describe their RCTs (O'Cathain et al., 2014b). Many of the journal articles described 'usual care' as the control arm in the RCT, indicating that the RCTs were at the pragmatic end of the spectrum. The qualitative research used with these RCTs focused much more on the feasibility and acceptability of the intervention, as well the trial conduct, outcomes, and outcome measurement.

Guidance for undertaking qualitative research alongside pragmatic RCTs is available (Oakley et al., 2006). In addition, published guidance for process evaluations undertaken alongside RCTs of complex interventions is highly relevant to the use of qualitative research with pragmatic RCTs (Moore et al., 2015). This latter guidance addresses both the feasibility/pilot phase of a study where the rationale is to improve the intervention and the RCT conduct, and the evaluation phase where the rationale is to explain the RCT results, although by far the main focus is on the latter phase. According to this guidance, the key functions of the process evaluation focus on the intervention: its mechanisms of impact, its implementation, and the context in which it operates. Context is extremely important for pragmatic RCTs because it can affect both the intervention implementation and the outcomes achieved. As discussed in Chapter 3, qualitative research can be used to explore all three functions of a process evaluation.

4.3 Feasibility, pilot, or exploratory RCTs

The MRC guidance on the development and evaluation of complex interventions recommends an early phase of assessing feasibility prior to a full evaluation (Craig et al., 2008). In this 'feasibility and pilot' phase, researchers can identify and address problems that could undermine the acceptability and delivery of the intervention or the conduct of the full RCT. This phase may result in researchers moving on to the next phase of a full RCT if problems identified are fixable, or returning to the development phase of a study if fundamental problems are identified with the intervention or the RCT conduct.

Offering a definition of this RCT type is difficult because researchers sometimes use the terms feasibility, pilot, and exploratory to describe the same type of study or RCT, while other researchers attempt to distinguish between these terms. Other terms may also be used, for example a 'formative' study as part of 'evidence-based planning' in preparation for an RCT (Behets et al., 2008). Eldridge et al. (2016) offer clarity to this area by identifying the territory as 'in preparation for an RCT'. Although they started from a position of mutually exclusive definitions of pilot and feasibility studies, they ended up documenting pilot studies as a subset of feasibility studies: a feasibility study asks whether something can be done; a pilot study may do the same but conducts a mini-version of part or all of the future full study.

The feasibility/pilot phase for a full RCT does not have to include an RCT. It can be

- qualitative, using interviews and non-participant observation to refine the intervention and its implementation,
- mixed methods, with qualitative research alongside a quantitative pretest–post-test study of the use of the intervention. The quantitative study can measure processes such as retention rates for the intervention and performance of the intervention in terms of improvements in interim outcomes,
- qualitative research or a process evaluation alongside an external pilot RCT. Here the feasibility study can address randomization processes, the recruitment rate for the full RCT, and retention in the intervention and control arms, as well as issues addressed in the other two designs.

4.3.1 Guidance for using qualitative research in feasibility studies for RCTs

Guidance is available for using qualitative research in feasibility studies for RCTs (O'Cathain et al., 2015). This guidance is summarized in Table 4.1. Some items in this guidance are as relevant to qualitative research undertaken alongside full RCTs as they are to the preparation phase for the full RCT. Items with specific relevance to the feasibility and pilot phase are the following.

- **Prioritizing uncertainties to be addressed:** At the feasibility phase of any study there are many uncertainties and researchers will need to consider where the most important uncertainties lie and use their limited resources of time, money, and manpower to address these. Returning to Chapter 3 can help to identify a long list of questions and uncertainties for the research team to prioritize in the context of their study. The aim of qualitative research with this type of RCT is improvement of the intervention and/or the RCT conduct in preparation for the full RCT.
- **Taking a 'dynamic' approach:** If a pilot RCT is included in the feasibility study, researchers may be tempted to view the qualitative research undertaken alongside it as a mini-version of the qualitative research undertaken alongside the full RCT. A different approach can be taken because the aim of the pilot RCT is not effectiveness measurement. The aim of the pilot RCT is to test whether enough participants can be recruited, whether retention rates are high enough for internal validity, etc. Taking a dynamic approach to qualitative data collection, where qualitative data is undertaken early and actions are taken based on it to improve the intervention or the conduct of the pilot RCT

Table 4.1 Guidance on using qualitative research in feasibility studies

Aspects of the feasibility study	Issues to consider
1. Research questions	a. When designing the feasibility study, consider the wide range of questions. Then consider those best addressed by qualitative research
	b. Prioritize the initial questions by identifying key uncertainties, whilst allowing for the possibility of emergent questions
	c. Consider the often overlooked questions, such as 'what is considered to be usual care?'
2. Design and data collection	a. Consider the range of qualitative methods that might be used to address the key feasibility questions, including dynamic or iterative approaches which allow learning from early qualitative research findings to be implemented before further qualitative research is undertaken as part of the feasibility study
	b. Select from a range of appropriate qualitative methods to address the feasibility questions and provide a rationale for the choices made; non-participant observation may be an important consideration
	c. Pay attention to diversity when sampling participants, groups, sites and stage of intervention
	d. Appreciate the difference between qualitative research and public and patient involvement
3. Analysis	a. Consider timing of analysis which might be in stages in a dynamic approach
	b. Many different approaches to analysis can be used, including framework, thematic and grounded theory-informed analysis
	c. Data can cover a breadth of issues but the analysis may focus on a few key issues
4. Team working	a. Have a qualitative researcher as part of the feasibility study design team
	b. Consider relationships between the qualitative researchers and the wider feasibility study team
	c. Consider who will make changes to the intervention or trial conduct
5. Reporting	a. Publish feasibility studies where possible because they help other researchers consider the feasibility of similar interventions or trials
	b. Describe the qualitative analysis and findings in detail
	c. Be explicit about the learning for a future trial or a similar body of interventions or generic learning for trials

Reproduced from O'Cathain A, et al. (2015) Maximising the impact of qualitative research in feasibility studies for randomised controlled trials: guidance for researchers. *Feasibility and Pilot Studies*, Volume 1, Article 32, while the pilot RCT is ongoing, is possible and recommended. This means that an assessment can be made of the impact of actions taken in response to the qualitative research, and further problems identified by later qualitative research, before the end of the feasibility study. An excellent example of this dynamic approach is Donovan et al's (2002) study of recruitment rates for an RCT where they use qualitative research to study recruitment practices in a pilot RCT. This team has continued to refine this approach and describe it as an intervention to improve the conduct of specific RCTs (Donovan et al., 2016).

- **Working in an integrated way:** The qualitative researchers and the RCT researchers may choose to work separately in the evaluation or full RCT phase (see Chapter 12). Concerns about integrated working between qualitative researchers and the team running the RCT are not relevant at the feasibility phase. The focus is on the whole team learning as much as possible to improve both the intervention and the RCT conduct before spending large amounts of resource on the full RCT. Integrated working, where qualitative researchers feed back findings to the whole team throughout the feasibility study can benefit this process (see Chapter 12).
- **Planning changes to the intervention or RCT conduct:** If the qualitative research is to have the desired impact on the intervention and the full RCT, it is important that plans are made to act on its findings. The people who can make changes should be present at meetings in the feasibility phase and sign up to taking actions. Careful timetabling may be needed to put changes in place for the full RCT, especially if changes are required to the intervention.
- **Reporting the findings:** Researchers may hesitate to publish feasibility studies, viewing them as important only to their planned full RCT. Researchers may also be concerned that journals with high impact factors will not publish feasibility studies or be unwilling to commit time to writing a publication because it cannot it is not seen as having the same impact as the full evaluation. Where possible, it is recommended that researchers publish this work because it helps other researchers to consider the feasibility of similar interventions or RCTs. Publications can maximize utility by being explicit about the learning for a future RCT, or a similar body of interventions, or for RCTs generally.

4.3.2 Challenges when using qualitative research at the feasibility phase

There are challenges to undertaking qualitative research at the feasibility/pilot phase of an evaluation:

1. **Funding:** It may be difficult to obtain funding to undertake feasibility studies and different components of studies may have to be funded from different sources over time.

2. **Using the dynamic approach in practice:** Little has been written about the practicalities of taking a dynamic approach to data collection and analysis of the qualitative research. Iterations of data collection and analysis of qualitative research are only possible in a pilot RCT of sufficient length. Speedy data collection and analysis is required, as well as adequate resource for this.
3. **Making decisions about what needs to be changed:** If problems are identified with the RCT conduct or the intervention, the team has to decide whether to take action on each of these. If one member of staff delivering the intervention or one patient using the intervention raises a problem, is that sufficient evidence to take action? Team communication and decision making will be needed to identify which problems need to be addressed and how (see Chapter 12).
4. **Prioritizing changes within limited resources:** Even when researchers are clear that changes are necessary to the RCT conduct or intervention, these can take time and money to instigate. These resources may not be available and the team will need to prioritize changes in the context of how much they cost. Planning can help here. In a pilot RCT and process evaluation of a website to increase adherence to medication in adults with cystic fibrosis (CFHealthHub, 2016), the team planned a time when the qualitative researchers would complete their first iteration of data collection and analysis and report findings to the wider team. The team developing the intervention allocated manpower for the time period after this feedback to make any necessary changes to the website before further qualitative research was then undertaken later in the pilot RCT.
5. **Publishing feasibility studies:** Researchers do publish qualitative research undertaken in feasibility studies for RCTs but may find it challenging to locate journals willing to publish it, or construct journal articles reporting this research. An open access journal called *Pilot and Feasibility Studies* has been established to publish these studies (BioMed Central, 2017). Informal templates may emerge over time that help future researchers to more easily write these journal articles. An example of a pilot RCT with embedded qualitative study is described in Box 4.1.

4.4 Cluster RCTs

In cluster RCTs, groups of people, such as families or communities, or people attending organizations such as schools, general practices, or hospitals, are randomized rather than individuals. Grant et al. (2013) offer a framework for designing and reporting process evaluations undertaken alongside cluster

Box 4.1 An example of a pragmatic pilot RCT with embedded qualitative study

Hubbard and colleagues (2016) undertook a pragmatic pilot RCT to assess whether cardiac rehabilitation was feasible and acceptable to promote exercise and recovery in post-surgical colorectal cancer survivors. Patients were referred to weekly classes in cardiac rehabilitation that were also attended by patients with cardiovascular disease. The RCT took place in a routine health setting and the intervention was compared with usual care in this setting. Forty-one patients participated in the RCT and quantitative data were collected on numbers consenting to participate in the RCT and numbers completing the intervention. Twenty-two patients with colorectal cancer, eight patients with cardiovascular disease, and 11 nursing and physiotherapy staff participated in a concurrent qualitative interview study. Qualitative data were analysed using framework analysis. Researchers identified that the intervention was both acceptable and feasible. A perceived benefit of the intervention was that it increased participants' confidence and motivation to exercise. A barrier to using the intervention was the time taken for patients to recover from surgery. The team recommended in the abstract of the journal article that a full RCT be undertaken.

Source: data from Hubbard, G., et al. (2016) Is referral of postsurgical colorectal cancer survivors to cardiac rehabilitation feasible and acceptable? A pragmatic pilot randomised controlled trial with embedded qualitative study. *BMJ Open*, Volume 6, Issue 1.

RCTs (summarized in Box 4.2). Although the focus of their framework is not exclusively on qualitative research, they are explicit about the roles qualitative research can take when used with this type of RCT. The authors acknowledge that there is no best way to design and undertake a process evaluation for a cluster RCT but that the process evaluation will depend on the specific cluster RCT and the resources available. They put forward a structure to understand

- trial delivery,
- intervention implementation over time,
- and how individuals respond to the intervention.

There is considerable overlap between this guidance and guidance for process evaluations more generally (Moore et al., 2015). The unique aspect of this guidance is that researchers need to pay attention to clusters and individuals

Box 4.2 Roles of qualitative research used alongside cluster RCTs

Explore recruitment of clusters and of individuals: Understanding why some clusters participate and others do not can help to interpret the generalizability of the RCT results. Understanding why some individuals participate and others not can help to identify bias and interpret the RCT results.
Explore intervention implementation at the cluster level and amongst individuals in the clusters: Understanding how the intervention is delivered in each cluster can draw attention to implementation difficulties or variation in implementation between clusters. This can help to interpret the RCT results. Understanding how clusters or individuals change their engagement or implementation over time can help to appreciate how the intervention will fare in routine practice if found to be effective in the RCT.
Explore how clusters and individuals within them respond to the intervention: This is similar to mechanisms of impact which is identified as a key function of process evaluations by Moore et al. (2015).
Explore how the intervention is embedded within routine health services: If staff delivering the new intervention can integrate this into their normal practice, this fares well for knowledge translation if it is found to be effective in the RCT and subsequently adopted for use in routine care. This concept is explored further in Chapter 6.
Explore variation in effectiveness between clusters: Understanding why some clusters show improvements in the primary outcome and others not can help to understand transferability of RCT results to different contexts. An example of this is described is Box 4.3.
Understand context: Clusters may be in different countries for example, and this wider context may affect how the intervention is implemented or the outcomes achieved. The example in Box 4.3 shows how a contextual issue of resource availability affected outcomes achieved in each cluster in an RCT.

Source: data from Grant, A., et al. (2013) Process evaluations for cluster randomised trials of complex interventions: a proposed framework for design and reporting. *Trials*, Issue 14, p. 15. doi: 10.1186/1745-6215-14-15.

associated with the RCT. For example, qualitative research can be used to explore variation between clusters (see Box 4.3). Although Grant et al. (2013) focus on intervention clusters they point out the importance of also understanding what occurs in control clusters.

Box 4.3 An example of qualitative research used with a cluster RCT—the Breastfeeding in Groups (BIG) Study

Hoddinott and colleagues (2010) undertook a cluster RCT in 14 localities in Scotland. Health professionals in the seven intervention localities were asked to increase group activities related to breastfeeding. The research team hypothesized that there would be differences between the intervention clusters. They carried out focus groups, interviews, and observations of breastfeeding groups during the RCT. Before conducting analysis of the outcomes of the RCT, they used the qualitative research to construct an explanatory model of factors contributing to the success or failure of the localities in delivering the intervention. The outcome of the RCT was null, with breastfeeding rates declining in three of the seven intervention localities. The model helped the researchers to explain these differences in outcomes between clusters by identifying problems with the leadership with some localities, the place where the group sessions were held, and a lack of resources in the clusters with declining breastfeeding rates.

Source: data from Hoddinott, P. et al. Why do interventions work in some places and not others: a breastfeeding support group trial. *Social Science & Medicine*, Volume 70, Issue 5, pp. 769–778. Copyright © 2009 Elsevier Ltd.

Challenges for the qualitative research include working with large numbers of clusters and balancing the focus on clusters and on individuals. Sometimes there are small numbers of clusters and all intervention clusters can be included in the qualitative research (see example in Box 4.3). Where there are large numbers of clusters, sampling is required for the qualitative research. A combination of diverse sampling in the qualitative research and a mixed methods approach at the cluster level may be required whereby the qualitative research facilitates design of a questionnaire which can be completed by all clusters. In terms of getting the balance right between spending resources on qualitative research on the cluster or on the individuals, research teams need to discuss priorities for the qualitative research at the planning stage of the mixed methods study.

Clusters can be allocated to intervention and control in parallel or in sequence in a stepped wedge design. There is increasing use of stepped wedge cluster RCTs in developed countries for the evaluation of educational interventions

(Beard et al., 2015). Qualitative research has been used with stepped wedge cluster RCTs and in ways that are similar to parallel cluster RCTs (Aoun et al., 2015). The sequencing of cross over from control to intervention over time can introduce challenges as changes occur in context over time. Qualitative research can be used to explore contextual changes over the time this type of RCT occurs.

4.5 N of 1 trials

N of 1 trials are cross-over studies in individuals that estimate the treatment effect on an individual patient and thereby facilitate individualized treatment. An individual is randomly assigned to using the intervention or control over different time periods on multiple occasions. N of 1 trials are useful for people with chronic conditions where treatment response is stable over time, the treatment offers an immediate effect, and the treatment has negligible carryover effects (Duan et al., 2013). They can also be useful for evaluating interventions in rare conditions. They have been used to test behavioural interventions as well as drugs (Sneihotta et al., 2012). Qualitative research has shown that this type of RCT can be acceptable to patients (Brookes et al., 2007).

There is no formal guidance on using qualitative research with this type of RCT. Nor is there enough published experience of using qualitative research with it to determine the challenges involved, although some researchers have offered reflections on it. Van Ness et al. (2016) consider how qualitative research can be used alongside N of 1 trials within a mixed methods study. They describe how qualitative research can be used to

- assess the trial conduct, for example, by interviewing participants about their perceptions of the effectiveness of the 'wash out' periods;
- explore participants' perceptions of benefits, to be considered alongside the quantitative outcome measures for each individual. Although Van Ness and colleagues cite concerns expressed by other scholars about using qualitative research to validate RCT findings, qualitative research can identify benefits and adverse issues that are not being measured in the RCT.

Because each patient is analysed separately in the RCT, it is best to view the qualitative research as a case study for each patient. A mixed methods analysis would place the quantitative and qualitative data for a single patient side by side in a matrix for comparison (see Chapter 11). Then the quantitative and qualitative data on each patient can be viewed as multiple case studies and pattern matching used to determine which types of patients are benefiting and why. This mixed methods approach can be useful at the feasibility and pilot phase of an evaluation when researchers are exploring the potential for an intervention to be effective. It can also useful at the implementation phase when interventions found to be effective on average are tested for effectiveness in individual patients.

4.6 Factorial RCTs

A factorial RCT is where two or more intervention comparisons are carried out simultaneously. A protocol for a mixed methods study which includes a 2×2 factorial RCT to compare the effectiveness of two interventions for improving the gait of children with cerebral palsy, and the effectiveness of combining the two therapies is described in Box 2.1 in Chapter 2. The team's concurrent qualitative research was an interview study with 18 parent and child dyads on two occasions. Another example, described in Chapter 9, Figure 9.1, is a factorial cluster RCT with four arms (Tonkin-Crine et al., 2014). Three of the arms received an intervention for acute cough consultations in general practice (intervention A, intervention B, and both interventions together). Qualitative interviews were undertaken with 62 patients in all three interventions arms, balancing sampling across the three arms. This suggests that a potential challenge of using qualitative research with this type of RCT is that larger samples may be required for any qualitative research, and comparison of qualitative research between arms in the qualitative analysis essential. There is no published guidance about the use of qualitative research alongside factorial RCTs.

4.7 New designs

Adaptive RCTs, where prospectively planned changes are made to the design based on ongoing outcome data as the RCT progresses, are of current interest. In sequential multiple assignment randomized trials (SMARTs), participants are initially randomized to one treatment option and then may be re-randomized at later points in the RCT to consider long-term outcomes (Moodie et al., 2016). There is no reason why qualitative research could not make a contribution alongside these designs, both to explore the intervention and to understand the implications of the conduct of these newer designs. To date, there is only a qualitative study of stakeholders' views of adaptive design rather than examples of qualitative research used with adaptive designs in practice (Dimairo et al., 2015).

4.8 Key points

- Qualitative research can be undertaken with explanatory RCTs but is more likely to be undertaken with pragmatic RCTs.
- Feasibility or pilot RCTs are different from full RCTs. When undertaking qualitative research, researchers can take a dynamic approach to data collection, feeding back findings to the team so that changes can be made to the pilot RCT conduct, and intervention during the feasibility pilot phase.
- Qualitative research undertaken alongside a cluster RCT needs to consider processes at the cluster and the individual level.
- Qualitative research can be used with N of 1 trials to contribute to understanding how best to individualize treatment at the implementation phase of an evaluation. Analysis of qualitative research will be different from that used in the context of other types of RCTs, focusing on multiple mixed methods case studies.
- Qualitative research used with factorial RCTs is likely to focus on how patients view two or more interventions in the RCT. This is likely to require a larger sample size than a RCT with one active arm, and comparison between intervention arms is likely at analysis.
- There appears to be little primary qualitative research undertaken with newer designs such as adaptive trials but this is likely to change in the future.

4.9 Questions to help you think about your study

- What type of RCT are you intending to undertake?
- What is the key issue to attend to when undertaking qualitative research with this type of RCT?

Further reading

Moore, G., Audrey, S., Barker, M., Bond, L., Bonell, C., Cooper, C., Hardeman, W., Moore, L., O'Cathain, A., Tannaze, T., Wight, D., Baird, J. (2015). Process evaluation of complex interventions. Medical Research Council guidance. *BMJ*, **350**, h1258. doi: 10.1136/bmj.h1258.

Grant, A., Treweek, S., Dreischulte, T., Foy, R., Guthrie, B. (2013). Process evaluations for cluster randomised trials of complex interventions: a proposed framework for design and reporting. *Trials*, **14**, 15. doi: 10.1186/1745-6215-14-15.

Chapter 5

Paradigms

Overview

Read this chapter to learn about different paradigms or 'world views' relevant to this endeavour, including

- Implicit post-positivism
- Participatory action research
- Transformative, e.g. community-based participatory research
- 'Dynamic'
- Realism
- Dialectical pluralism

5.1 Introduction

A paradigm is a world view held by members of a research community. It is a set of beliefs that determine what humans can know and how best to undertake research to generate knowledge. It shapes how any research is undertaken and how its quality is judged (see Chapter 13 for details about assessing the quality of qualitative research undertaken with RCTs). In mixed methods evaluations that combine qualitative research and RCTs, the implicit paradigm is often post-positivism. There are alternative paradigms such as participatory action research and realist evaluation. The status of the qualitative research within a mixed methods evaluation may depend on the paradigm adopted. It can also be the case that researchers undertaking the qualitative research adopt a different philosophical stance from those undertaking the RCT. Therefore it is important to have team discussions about paradigms throughout a mixed methods evaluation to understand the variety of stances within the team. The focus of this chapter is on the range of paradigms researchers can adopt and some of the challenges researchers can face when combining qualitative research and RCTs within different paradigms.

5.2 RCTs and qualitative research—different paradigms?

RCTs are favoured by researchers who believe that measuring the effectiveness of an intervention in an unbiased way is the most important contribution to be made to knowledge about health and health care. These researchers are aware of the impossibility of eliminating bias, and therefore of being certain about their results, but are nonetheless driven by the importance of removing as much bias as possible through randomisation and blinding when measuring effectiveness. Researchers leading RCTs of complex interventions rather than of drugs are increasingly aware of the importance of social relationships and context to the question of effectiveness. They welcome non-experimental methods and qualitative research to understand complexity and how context shapes effectiveness. An appropriate label for this paradigm is 'post-positivism', or more accurately 'implicit post-positivism' because these researchers are rarely explicit about the paradigm they work within when seeking funding or publishing journal articles because it is a dominant paradigm in health evaluation currently.

Qualitative research is associated with the paradigm of constructivism or interpretivism where researchers believe that human beings construct reality. That is, they believe that there is no single external truth but rather a number of truths perceived by different human beings. Questions that tend to be important to researchers working in this paradigm relate to the complexity of human actions such as why health practitioners or patients act as they do, or how patients experience a health condition. Within this paradigm, researchers are not interested in bias reduction but on the importance of understanding the role of researchers on the research they undertake. These researchers practice reflexivity where they reflect on the effect they as researchers are having, or have had, on the data collection, analysis and interpretation of their research. Although this paradigm is commonly associated with qualitative research, it is also the case that qualitative research can be undertaken within many other paradigms, including post-positivism.

The 'paradigm wars' occurred in the 1980s when there was a belief that quantitative and qualitative research could not be undertaken in the same study because each method could only be undertaken within a different paradigm. This belief is no longer dominant within many health research communities. Mixed methods scholars have described how qualitative and quantitative research can be undertaken within a range of paradigms (Bryman, 1998; Creswell and Plano Clark, 2007; Morgan, 2007), and mixed methods evaluation within paradigms such as post-positivism, constructivism, pragmatism, and transformative (Mertens and Tarsilla, 2015). In the field of evaluation, Greene et al. (2001) view a mixed methods approach to evaluation as necessary because evaluation is often undertaken in natural settings and this complexity requires bringing together different ways of knowing. They propose a dialectic stance that promotes dialogue between two very different ways of thinking about research—quantitative and qualitative—so that insights emerge from these differences. The range of paradigms within which qualitative research and RCTs can be undertaken, and indeed have been undertaken, are detailed in Section 5.3.

5.3 Paradigms for combining qualitative research and RCTs

5.3.1 Implicit post-positivism

As described in Section 5.2, researchers are not always explicit about their paradigms. When combining qualitative research and RCTs, researchers leading the RCT usually work within a post-positivist paradigm and qualitative researchers may adopt any number of paradigms including post-positivism. The RCT is viewed as the most important component of the evaluation, or even viewed as *the* evaluation, and the qualitative research is welcomed as a junior partner as long as it does not interfere with the RCT in any way. Taking an 'implicit' approach may be problem free or, because the RCT is dominant, the qualitative research may be subsumed within its paradigm and conflicts may occur around different values and beliefs held by different researchers in the team (Simons, 2007). Three problems can occur by adopting this philosophical stance:

1. **Low status of qualitative research:** Because the qualitative research takes an enhancing role within the mixed methods evaluation (Popay and Williams, 1998), rather than being viewed as integral to the evaluation, the epistemological stance of the researchers leading the RCT can dominate (Song et al., 2010). This can lead to the evaluation being viewed as an 'RCT with add-ons' where the qualitative research is one such add-on. This in turn can lead to the qualitative research being under resourced and disregarded (O'Cathain et al., 2014a).
2. **Tensions between team members:** There may be tensions between the RCT researchers who value statistical generalizability, objectivity, predetermined protocols, and control of the context in which the research takes place and the qualitative researchers who value more inductive, flexible approaches to research with a focus on context and subjectivity. If the values of the RCT researchers dominate then qualitative researchers may be asked to increase their sample sizes, undertake probability sampling where this is not the best

approach, and adhere to specified procedures throughout their study when an iterative flexible approach would be more useful (O'Cathain et al., 2014a).

3. **Damage to the qualitative research:** Giddings (2006) expresses concern that mixed methods research is simply 'post-positivism in drag' and results in the loss of the strengths of qualitative research. A few decades ago there were concerns that the 'RCT paradigm' could damage qualitative research, with it likened to a wolf devouring the qualitative research (Popay and Williams, 1998). More recently, Hesse-Biber (2012) has expressed concerns that RCT researchers emphasize the objectivity of researchers who must desist from allowing their values to contaminate the research environment, and that this can shape the way in which the qualitative research is conducted. She also expresses concern about the dominance of the RCT limiting the types of questions addressed by the qualitative research, and imposing values on it that are more important to quantitative research.

Problems do not necessarily occur where an implicit post-positivist stance is taken. There may be methodological understanding between team members who value the diversity of methods within the evaluation. Problems can also be prevented by holding team discussions at the planning stage of the study to share beliefs and values held by different team members, and how they can be accommodated (see Chapter 14).

5.3.2 Participatory action research

Participatory action research involves collaboration between researchers and participants, and engages in cyclical processes of action–feedback–action–feedback. Implementation science, with its focus on implementing change in a wide variety of settings in the real world of clinical practice, and community-based public health evaluation with its focus on empowering communities to make sustained change, have been open to participatory action approaches to evaluation. Researchers undertaking RCTs in these fields are acutely aware of the complex environments in which they are testing interventions for health improvement and understand the need to learn from people embedded in those contexts through iterations of research. These researchers are willing to take a different world view of evaluation shaped by what they want to achieve: sustained change in the real world.

Leykum et al. (2009) have proposed integrating participatory action research with an RCT in a way that plays to the strengths of both, balancing the need for standardization of an intervention within an RCT with adaptation of aspects of the intervention at a local level to help it work in different contexts. That is, the view of the intervention is that it is not fixed but has fixed and flexible aspects to it (Hawe et al., 2004), allowing participation from local sites to adapt the flexible aspects to their context. Reflection on implementation of the intervention throughout the RCT can result in changes made at local levels to accommodate local context. This approach may require changes to traditional RCT designs, such as each site participating in the RCT being allowed to measure additional endpoints. Qualitative methods can be used to facilitate participation and be used in more traditional ways to explore implementation of the intervention and the RCT. An example of a participatory 'informed by the principles of action research' (Hoddinott et al., 2012, p. 2) is described in Box 5.1).

Box 5.1 Example of participatory research used to inform a full RCT

Hoddinott and colleagues (2012) used a participatory approach to design, deliver and implement an intervention aiming to improve breastfeeding among women from disadvantaged areas. The intervention was telephone support from a feeding support team integrated into routine postnatal hospital ward care. The study consisted of a pilot RCT and a mixed methods process evaluation focusing on the study acceptability, feasibility and intervention fidelity from the perspectives of women and health practitioners. A participatory approach informed by the principles of action research was used to design, implement and evaluate the intervention. The rationale for this approach was that the intervention and the RCT had to be workable in routine care because of the low level of resource in this part of the health care system. The study was undertaken in preparation for a full RCT. A steering group of practitioners, managers, and researchers met over the course of the study to design the study and intervention and consider implementation of both the intervention and the RCT. The steering group members discussed issues about the pilot RCT such as how best to randomize women, and reasons for problems with recruitment. Meetings were audio recorded and analysed with other data using framework analysis.

Source: data from Hoddinott, P et al. (2012) 'Process evaluation for the FEeding Support Team (FEST) randomised controlled feasibility trial of proactive and reactive telephone support for breastfeeding women living in disadvantaged areas'. *BMJ Open*, 2012;2:e001039. doi: 10.1136/bmjopen-2012-001039.

5.3.3 Transformative paradigm

In a transformative paradigm the focus is on enhancing lives of marginalized members of society (Mertens and Tarsilla, 2015). Community-based participatory research is often undertaken within this paradigm. This is where the community is involved in decisions about how to implement the intervention and research within their community. Trickett (2011) describes the world view of community-based participatory research as where the community is the unit of interest to the research; there is community involvement in decision making about the intervention; community empowerment is part of the process; and a key focus is sustainability of benefits from the intervention after the RCT. However, Trickett is not convinced that these strengths can occur in practice when an RCT is used within the evaluation. Instead, he expresses concern that the RCT determines the actions taken within the evaluation and only a limited number of decisions can be taken in collaboration with communities. Goodkind et al. (2016) share some of his concerns about the challenges faced when undertaking qualitative research and an RCT within this paradigm but list a number of studies that have done so successfully. They describe the importance of a long and resourced planning phase for the evaluation. They also describe in detail the challenges of combining qualitative research and an RCT within community-based participatory research when testing the effectiveness of a collaboratively developed community-based social support intervention to reduce mental health disparities among refugee adults in the USA. Challenges included community members not seeing the necessity of an RCT because some of them had experienced the intervention and believed it worked, and interviewers wishing to help community members participating in the RCT. Solutions to address these challenges included random assignment of RCT participants at a public meeting, and having a clear protocol for offering help to community members and documenting any help given. An example of a community-based participatory approach is described in Box 5.2. Qualitative research can be used as part of the participatory infrastructure (as in the example in Box 5.2) and/or as part of a process evaluation.

5.3.4 'Dynamic' approach

A dynamic approach is not a formal paradigm, but is a term that has been used to describe a form of iterative action research where qualitative research is undertaken to improve recruitment for a specific RCT (Donovan et al., 2002). Here, the RCT has been described as embedded within qualitative research and this approach. Non-participant observation and qualitative interviews are used to explore how staff recruit participants for the RCT and how patients

Box 5.2 Example of community-based participatory approach including an RCT

Balcazar and colleagues (2009) undertook a pragmatic RCT of health education classes and contact with community health workers to prevent cardiovascular disease. The intervention was aimed at a 'hard to reach' group of Mexican American adults in a US–Mexico border community. Participants in the RCT were 328 Hispanic adults aged 30–75 years with at least one risk factor for cardiovascular disease (overweight, smoking, high cholesterol, diabetic, or hypertensive). The community-based participatory research included a forum of community group representatives, three focus groups with community members (men, women, community stakeholders) and development of an advisory council for the study. The key driver for using this approach appeared to be ensuring the RCT was feasible in the local context through developing two way communication between researchers and the community, and disseminating RCT baseline data to show the community the need for the intervention. The researchers felt they obtained 'buy in' from the community for the RCT but recognized the challenge of community-based participatory approach in the context of needing to follow a rigid RCT protocol.

Source: data from Balcazar, H. (2009). 'Use of community-based participatory research to disseminate baseline results from a cardiovascular disease randomized community trial for Mexican Americans living in a U.S.-Mexico border community'. *Education for Health*, Volume 22, Issue 3, p. 279. Copyright © 2009 Elsevier.

view the recruitment process. Anonymized feedback is given to the RCT team during the RCT and changes are made to recruitment procedures based on this qualitative research. Further iterations of qualitative research can be undertaken throughout the RCT. Recruitment rates are measured over time to see if changes made to recruitment processes result in increased recruitment rates. Although this approach was originally used in a feasibility and pilot trial (Donovan et al., 2002), it can also be used in full RCTs experiencing poor recruitment. The approach has been conceptualized as a complex intervention for improving RCT recruitment rates—the QuinteT Recruitment intervention (Donovan et al., 2016). The term 'dynamic' is not used to describe it in later publications. Describing it as a paradigm is not quite right but the way in which action is taken during the RCT in iterative cycles identifies a set of values and beliefs related to a paradigm.

5.3.5 **Realism**

Researchers undertaking RCTs have been criticized for focusing on the question 'is this intervention effective' rather than considering how interventions work, for whom, and under what circumstances. Bonell et al. (2012) propose that 'realist RCTs' focus on refining generalizable intervention theory while preserving the high internal validity of the RCT for measuring effectiveness. This occurs by focusing on mechanisms of change, undertaking multiple RCTs across different contexts to test how intervention effects vary with context, making use of a range of qualitative and quantitative methods, and focusing on building and validating program theories which show how interventions interact with context to produce outcomes. Realist RCTs are proposed as more appropriate for public health interventions because the effectiveness of these complex interventions is likely to vary in different contexts. The RCT is one of many methods used within the evaluation rather than the main priority, because the focus on context and theory refinement increases the perceived value of the other methods within the evaluation, especially the qualitative research (although the terminology 'realist RCT' does not quite communicate the lack of dominance of the RCT in such a paradigm). A challenge to this approach is that it is likely to be expensive as a series of co-ordinated RCTs is required, although the authors argue that this would be a better way of spending resource than the current uncoordinated large numbers of RCTs being undertaken within a post-positivist paradigm. Not all scholars agree that RCTs can be undertaken within a realist paradigm because RCTs are so grounded in post-positivism and recommend that Bonell et al. (2012) relabel their approach as 'theory-informed RCT' (Marchal et al., 2013). An example of how a realist RCT might work is shown in Box 5.3.

5.3.6 **Dialectical pluralism**

Qualitative and RCT researchers within a mixed methods evaluation may adopt different paradigms. Johnson and Schoonenboom (2015) propose the meta-paradigm of dialectical pluralism as a way of improving RCTs in health. This stance views reality as plural and recommends conversation between different team members and methods to generate knowledge. The concept of reflexivity is important so that researchers can have ongoing discussions with each other and wider stakeholders, respect differences, and learn from tensions and differences.

Box 5.3 An example of a realist RCT of a public health intervention to reduce aggression in schools

Jamal and colleagues (2015) describe a working example of a realist RCT of a school-wide intervention to reduce bullying. This consisted of a cluster RCT in 40 schools and integral process evaluation using diaries completed by intervention deliverers, researcher observations, interviews with staff, students, and intervention deliverers, surveys to measure satisfaction and implementation of the intervention, and in-depth case studies based on qualitative research in a sample of intervention schools. They describe how they will use emerging findings from the integral process evaluation to refine and generate a priori hypotheses before collecting quantitative follow-up data. They show how they plan to test these hypotheses using a combination of process and outcome quantitative analyses. These results will then be used to refine the theory of change. They propose that innovation is necessary in RCT procedures, for example that protocols allow for some adaptation of plans over time.

Source: data from Jamal, F., et al. (2015). 'The three stages of building and testing midlevel theories in a realist RCT: a theoretical and methodological case-example'. *Trials*, Issue 16, p. 466. Copyright © Jamal et al. 2015.

5.4 Key points

- Although evaluations which combine qualitative research and RCTs are often undertaken within a paradigm of implicit post-positivism, they can be undertaken within other paradigms which increase the status of the qualitative research within the evaluation, for example participatory and realist approaches.

5.5 Questions to help you think about your study

- What do you value in your research?
- What do you believe about truth and how best to generate knowledge?
- Do your team members share these values and beliefs?

- How are different sets of values and beliefs in your team affecting your evaluation?
- What conversations can occur to resolve differences that are causing problems, or maximise the value of these differences to learn more about the topic under study?

Further reading

Some researchers struggle to engage with paradigms. David Morgan offers a clear and sophisticated discussion about the different meanings of the word paradigms and paradigms for mixed methods research. Mertens and Tarsilla (2016) present an excellent reflection on paradigms for mixed methods evaluation (although not specifically those including an RCT).

Morgan, D.L. (2007). Paradigms lost and pragmatism regained methodological implications of combining qualitative and quantitative methods. *Journal of Mixed Methods Research*, **1**(1), pp. 48–76. doi: 10.1177/2345678906292462.

Mertens, D.M., Tarsilla, M. (2015). Mixed-methods evaluation. In: Hesse-Biber, S.N., Johnson, R.B. (eds) *The Oxford Handbook of Multimethod and Mixed Methods Research Inquiry*. Oxford Library of Psychology. Oxford: Oxford University Press. pp. 426–446.

Chapter 6

Theories underpinning the intervention

Overview

Read this chapter to learn about

- The role of theory in generating evidence of effectiveness
- The relationship between qualitative research and theories
- Examples of theories or frameworks of theories relevant to mixed methods evaluation in health research
- Challenges of using theory in this context

6.1 Introduction

Researchers have theories about how the interventions they are evaluating achieve effectiveness (mechanisms of action) and how best to implement them in complex environments. It is recommended that these theories are made explicit, either by drawing on existing theories from organizational, psychological, improvement science, or sociological research, or displaying programme theories specific to the intervention that show the proposed causal pathways from content of intervention to long-term outcomes. These theories can shape the research questions, sampling, data collection, analysis, interpretation, and reporting of any qualitative research undertaken with RCTs. Some relevant theories are introduced, with examples of how researchers have used them with qualitative research and RCTs.

6.2 The role of theory in generating evidence of effectiveness

Davidoff et al. (2015) in their article on demystifying theory distinguish two types of theory relevant to generating evidence of effectiveness:

1. 'Mid-range' or 'middle range' or 'big' or 'formal' theories which offer frameworks for developing and understanding complex interventions, e.g. Diffusion of Innovations and Normalization Process Theory.

2. 'Programme' or 'small' or 'informal' theories which are specific to an intervention and are usually described in a logic model showing the components of an intervention that address different aspects of the relevant health problem and how they lead to intermediate outcomes and primary outcomes.

These two types of theory can be used in combination, and a number of mid-range theories can be used in combination or alone.

Theory can help to

- identify the problems that the intervention will attempt to address;
- design an appropriate intervention;
- design an evaluation which measures and explores relevant processes and outcomes;
- optimize RCT procedures such as recruitment;
- identify how an intervention works—its mechanisms of action;
- identify aspects of context that support effectiveness of the intervention;
- understand the RCT results;
- pay attention to feasibility of the intervention in routine care and optimize the chance of RCT findings being used in practice after an intervention has been shown to be effective;
- help replication of an effective intervention outside the original context that it was tested.

6.3 The relationship between qualitative research and theory

Qualitative research can be used to develop and refine theories underpinning interventions and their implementation (May et al., 2011). Alternatively, theories can shape how qualitative research is undertaken when used with RCTs.

- At the development phase of an evaluation, qualitative research can support the design of a theory-informed intervention by identifying the most important aspects of a mid-range theory for the specific intervention or how they operate in a specific context (see the example in Box 6.1).
- At the feasibility phase of an evaluation, qualitative research can identify tacit components of the intervention, mechanisms of action observed or perceived by those delivering and receiving the intervention, and causal

Box 6.1 Example of using organizational theory in a qualitative interview study undertaken prior to a cluster RCT

Bosch and colleagues (2016) undertook a qualitative interview study with emergency department staff in Australia prior to developing an intervention to increase uptake of evidence-based practice for the management of mild head injury. They planned to evaluate the intervention in a cluster RCT, with emergency departments as clusters. They used qualitative research to develop the intervention, interviewing nine directors, 20 doctors, and 13 nurses in 13 emergency departments. They drew on a range of organizational theories, and a conceptual model of those theories, in the qualitative research and the whole programme of research. Their rationale for focusing on organizational theory was that emergency departments are complex and unique organizations. They used this organizational level theory in complement with psychological theory because they believed that both organizational and individual level factors affected management of minor head injury. Organizational theories were selected by a multidisciplinary group within the research team based on their perceived relevance to emergency departments. The researchers used these theories in their topic guide for the qualitative interviews, and used the conceptual model of Diffusion of Innovation as a framework for their analysis and organization of results within their published article. The qualitative research was used to gain an understanding of the relative importance of these organizational factors in this setting and inform the components of a new intervention to address important modifiable factors. The researchers plan to further use these theories in their mixed methods process evaluation alongside the cluster RCT to understand the extent to which different aspects of the intervention were effective and why. They perceived that the qualitative research reported here would help them to explain the results of their future RCT because of the understanding it gave of the context in which the intervention would operate.

Source: data from Bosch, M., et al. (2016) The many organisational factors relevant to planning change in emergency care departments: A qualitative study to inform a cluster randomised controlled trial aiming to improve the management of patients with mild traumatic brain injuries. *PLoS ONE* February 4, 2016, doi:/10.1371/0148091. © 2016 Bosch et al.

Box 6.2 Example of using behavioural theory within a process evaluation alongside an RCT

Curran and colleagues (2013) used the Theoretical Domains Framework (TDF) to design a retrospective 'theory-based process evaluation'. This is an example of qualitative research being used after an RCT (see Section 2.3.4 in Chapter 2). The team had undertaken an RCT of The Canadian CT Head Rule, an intervention to help clinicians in emergency departments make decisions regarding the use of computed tomography in adult patients with minor head injury. The RCT was null which was surprising given that the same type of intervention had been shown to be successful in reducing the use of another diagnostic test in the same emergency departments. The team used the TDF to understand emergency physicians' responses to the intervention. Telephone interviews were undertaken with eight physicians from four of the six intervention sites in the RCT. The semi-structured interview guide used in the telephone interviews was based on the 12 domains from the TDF. The TDF was also used as a coding framework when analysing the interview transcripts, with 11 of the 12 domains useful for exploring barriers to the intervention. Content analysis was undertaken to code transcript content to each domain. Some domains of the TDF were identified as highly relevant to the failure of the intervention.

Source: data from Curran, J.A., et al. 'Understanding the Canadian adult CT head rule trial: use of the theoretical domains frameworks for process evaluation'. *Implementation Science*, Issue 8, p. 25.

pathways that have not been considered. This can help to develop the logic model which displays the programme theory underpinning the intervention (O'Cathain et al., 2013).

- During the full RCT, qualitative research can be used alone or within a process evaluation to explicitly explore the theory in terms of how mechanisms of action occurred in practice, how the intervention implementation aligned with theory, and how context impacted on causal pathways (Moore et al., 2015). See examples in Boxes 6.2 and 6.3.

The components of a theory or set of theories can shape the qualitative research in terms of

- identifying specific research questions;
- directing sampling decisions;

Box 6.3 Using Normalization Process Theory with a nested qualitative study alongside an RCT of collaborative care

Coupe and colleagues (2014) undertook a process evaluation alongside an RCT of collaborative care for managing patients with depression in primary care in the UK. They decided to re-analyse their data using the Normalization Process Theory to identify barriers and facilitators to the successful implementation of their intervention. They interviewed all 11 case managers and senior supervisors involved in delivering the intervention across three sites, and a purposive sample of 15 GPs whose practices participated in the trial. They conducted a thematic analysis and then undertook a further theory-driven analysis guided by the four constructs of Normalization Process Theory. They identified that GPs had limited understanding of the intervention and that there was little communication between them and the case managers. Organizational change was required to enhance collaboration. The researchers reported value in taking this approach to analysis.

Source: data from Coupe, N., et al. (2014) 'Facilitating professional liaison in collaborative care for depression in UK primary care; a qualitative study utilising normalisation process theory'. *BMC Family Practice*, Issue 15, p. 78. doi: 10.1186/1471-2296-15-78.

- identifying questions for data collection tools such as topic guides and observation sheets;
- offering a framework for the analysis of qualitative data;
- framing presentation of the qualitative findings.

The examples in Boxes 6.1–6.4 display some of these impacts of theory on the qualitative research used with RCTs.

6.4 Examples of theories

Interventions may be aimed at individual behaviours of health professionals, patients or the general population, or at organizations. There are numerous mid-range theories available for each of these scenarios and it can be difficult to choose between them. Fortunately, researchers have undertaken reviews of behaviour change and organizational theories and developed frameworks which bring together key domains of multiple theories. Key examples of theories and frameworks used with qualitative research and RCTs are explored in this section.

6.4.1 Behaviour change theory—the 'Theoretical Domains Framework'

The Theoretical Domains Framework is a consensus of the key theoretical constructs of behaviour change relevant to the implementation of evidence-based practice (Cane et al., 2012). It integrates 33 behaviour change theories into a more accessible structure. The 12 theoretical domains that explain behaviour change are (1) knowledge, (2) skills, (3) social/professional role and identity, (4) beliefs about capabilities, (5) beliefs about consequences, (6) motivation and goals, (7) memory, attention and decision processes, (8) environmental context and resources, (9) social influences, (10) emotion regulation, (11) behavioural regulation, and (12) nature of the behaviour. The Theoretical Domains Framework has been used to develop interventions for evaluation in RCTs and understand their implementation within RCTs. An example of its use in a retrospective qualitative process evaluation is described in Box 6.2.

6.4.2 The organizational theory framework 'Diffusion of Innovation'

Greenhalgh et al. (2004) considered how to deliver and sustain innovations in health services, where innovations are similar to complex interventions evaluated in RCTs. They undertook a systematic review of literature from a wide variety of disciplines including sociology, psychology, organization, and management. They identified the main determinants of diffusion, dissemination, and implementation of interventions in organizations. These determinants were numerous, acting at multiple levels including the innovation, the individuals adopting it, the system or organization, and the outer context. Examples of aspects of the innovation include compatibility with adopters' values and norms, and risk in terms of the degree of uncertainty of obtaining outcomes. Figure 3 in their paper summarizes the complex framework. An example of using this framework in a qualitative study undertaken before a full RCT is described in Box 6.1). It has also been used to consider variation in recruitment to a diagnostic test in general practices participating in a pragmatic cluster RCT (McMullen et al., 2015). In this last paper, qualitative data were analysed retrospectively using the model of Diffusion of Innovations rather than the model being used during collection of the qualitative data.

6.4.3 **Normalization Process Theory**

Normalization Process Theory focuses on the factors that help or hinder a complex intervention, health technology, or organizational innovation to become normal within routine practice (May et al. 2011). It can be used to consider the development and optimization of the RCT procedures as well as the intervention (Murray et al. 2010). Its focus on implementation when designing the intervention can help to prevent the development and evaluation of interventions that will not be implemented in the real world. There are four main components to Normalization Process Theory:

- *coherence* (or sense-making) encompasses whether the intervention makes sense to and is perceived to be of value to the relevant participants, and whether it fits with the goals and activities of the organization;
- *cognitive participation* (or engagement) considers whether participants will be prepared to invest in the new intervention;
- *collective action* (work done to enable the intervention to happen) asks what effect the intervention will have on current work, and whether it is consistent with existing practices; and
- *reflexive monitoring* (formal and informal appraisal of the benefits and costs of the intervention) asks how participants perceive the intervention once it has been in place for a while.

A systematic review of the use of Normalization Process Theory identified 29 studies that had used it as part of an evaluation (McEvoy et al., 2014). It has mainly being used within qualitative research to study the implementation of complex interventions that introduce a new way of working in health care settings. It has been used to inform the RCT or the intervention design, to generate research questions for fieldwork, to create tools for investigating implementation, and to act as an organizing framework for qualitative analysis and reporting of findings. It has broad appeal in that it has been used by researchers in different countries, different disciplines and for different types of interventions. McEvoy et al. (2014) have developed a helpful resource of examples. A further example is described in Box 6.3.

6.4.4 **RE-AIM**

RE-AIM (Reach, Effectiveness, Adoption, Implementation, and Maintenance) was introduced in the context of health promotion interventions in the USA (Glasgow et al., 1999). The five dimensions of the model or framework were proposed as key to considering the population-based impact of an intervention in contrast to a narrow focus on efficacy. Reach relates to the percentage of

Box 6.4 Example of the planned use of RE-AIM within a process evaluation alongside an RCT

Liu and colleagues (2016) plan to undertake an RCT of family-led rehabilitation after stroke in India. They describe their planned process evaluation to be undertaken alongside the RCT. They are interested in the translation of the RCT evidence in the real world, in particular the scalability and sustainability of the intervention after the evaluation. They used two theoretical frameworks, one of which was RE-AIM, because of its emphasis on real world implementation. The framework was used to identify the key questions for the mixed methods process evaluation. Semi-structured interviews with patients, carers, and staff were planned to obtain their views on mechanisms of action, how the intervention could be rolled out, and expectations of the intervention after the RCT. The framework would also shape the analysis, where the plan was to triangulate the qualitative and quantitative findings within different aspects of the framework.

Source: data from Liu, H., et al. 'Protocol for process evaluation of a randomised controlled trial of family-led rehabilitation post stroke (ATTEND) in India'. *BMJ Open*, Volume 6, Issue 9.

the target group that uses the intervention; efficacy to the size of effect; adoption to the proportion of organizations that would use the intervention in the real world; implementation to the extent to which the intervention was implemented as planned; and maintenance to the extent to which the intervention was sustained by individuals and organizations over time. An example of its planned use in a mixed methods process evaluation is described in Box 6.4.

6.4.5 Programme theory

Not all interventions are based on formal theory. In these cases it is recommended that researchers articulate assumptions about which components of an intervention produce which effects. Moore et al. (2015) recommend constructing a logic model, which is a diagram of the relationships between an intervention's components, intermediate outcomes and final health outcomes (Kellogg Foundation, 2004). A case has also been made for constructing a logic model of how an intervention can contribute to harm as well as benefit (Bonell et al., 2014). Qualitative research can be used during intervention development and play a part in constructing the logic model by identifying stakeholders' views of how they think the intervention will produce effect. Qualitative research can also be used within a process evaluation to identify support for, or breakdowns in, the proposed causal chains, additional aspects of the logic model, and challenges to assumptions documented within the logic model.

6.5 Challenges of using theory

6.5.1 Selecting the 'right' theory

The development of frameworks that bring together a range of theoretical constructs is a helpful addition to the literature so that researchers do not have to attempt to select one of 40 psychological or organizational theories. Selection of frameworks or theories will depend on the overarching aim of the intervention. For example, if researchers value the utility of their intervention in the real world, then the Normalization Process Theory may be a useful candidate for consideration. These frameworks and theories are not in competition with each other and a number of them may appear to offer helpful insights for the same study. It is interesting to consider Bosch et al. (2016) approach to identifying the 'right' theory for their study (see Box 6.1). They used both organizational and psychological theory and acknowledge that Normalization Process Theory and theories around team working were also relevant. They drew on a range of organizational level theories, and a framework that incorporated a range of theories, rather than a single theory. Bosch et al. (2016) display good practice by offering transparency about their process for considering the range of potential theories and the rationale for selecting the theories they decided to use. This good practice could be used more often than it is (McEvoy et al., 2014). It is recommended that researchers are transparent about the process and justification for selecting the theories and frameworks they have chosen to use.

6.5.2 Open data collection

A strength of qualitative research is that it uses open and often broad questions to allow interviewees to discuss issues of importance to them. Using a framework as the only approach to data collection, and then undertaking content analysis for each construct of the framework, may lead to blinkered thinking. Starting the interviews or observations in the qualitative research from a broad perspective and then moving to using a framework of theoretical constructs within data collection may offer a way of remaining open to understanding the extent to which the framework captures key issues.

6.5.3 Fit between the theory and the qualitative research

A selected theory is unlikely to fit the qualitative data perfectly and researchers will need to take a flexible approach to analysis and reporting (McEvoy et al.,

2014). Some domains of a theory will not be as relevant as others for some studies (McMullen et al., 2015; McEvoy et al., 2014). For example, two components of Normalization Process Theory were found to be more relevant to the planning stage of a study (Coherence and Cognitive Participation) and the other two to the experiences of implementing the intervention (Collective Action and Reflexive Monitoring) (McEvoy et al., 2014). Theories may also need to be extended to accommodate the full range of themes identified within the qualitative data (McMullen et al., 2015; McEvoy et al., 2014). A theory is only useful if it offers a good fit to the data and helps researchers to develop insights about their intervention and its implementation. If researchers sense at any point that they are missing important issues in their data collection, or shoe horning their data to fit the theory during the analysis of the qualitative data, then they will need to review the appropriateness of the framework or theory they are using.

6.5.4 Understanding the constructs of a theory

Understanding the constructs of a theory may not be straightforward (McEvoy et al., 2014) and applying the theory may require team discussion of the meaning of constructs, and double coding by different team members so that the analysts are confident about the application of the theory to the qualitative data.

6.6 Key points

- There are two types of theory relevant here: mid-range theory and programme theory.
- There are theories and frameworks of theoretical constructs available that can help researchers to understand more about the intervention and its implementation while preparing for an RCT or during the RCT (e.g., Theoretical Domains Framework, Diffusion of Innovations, Normalization Process Theory).
- Theories can shape the research questions, data collection, analysis, interpretation and reporting of the qualitative research.
- In the absence of a mid-range theory, programme theory specific to the intervention can be used. Even if a mid-range theory is used, it is helpful for the whole team to construct a logic model of how they expect different components of the intervention to affect processes and outcomes.
- A flexible approach to the application of theory is recommended.

6.7 Questions to help you think about your study

- Is your intervention intended to change the behaviour of individuals, organizations or both?
- How important is thinking about the implementation in the real world as you design and evaluate your intervention?
- Which mid-range theories might be relevant to your intervention?
- How does your theory translate into a logic model?
- How will this theory affect your qualitative study in terms of data collection, analysis and interpretation?
- What insights has your qualitative research generated about your intervention theory?

Further reading

Although Davidoff et al. (2015) wrote about theory in the context of improvement science, it is highly relevant to the use of qualitative research with RCTs:

Davidoff, F., Dixon-Woods, M., Leviton, L., Michie, S. (2015). Demystifying theory and its use in improvement. *BMJ Quality and Safety*, **24**(3), pp. 228–238. doi: 10.1136/bmjqs-2014-003627.

Part 2

Practical guidance for using qualitative research with RCTs

Chapter 7

Writing a proposal

Overview

Read this chapter to learn about writing a proposal for the qualitative research with a RCT:

- Types of proposals researchers need to write
- Existing guidance on writing proposals
- Detailed guidance for writing a research proposal in this context
- Challenges and potential solutions

When researchers plan to undertake qualitative research alongside a pilot or full RCT they write a proposal to apply for funding, seek ethical approval, or as part of their PhD studies. These proposals can be published in journals. Drabble et al. (2014) have published guidance for writing a proposal for the qualitative research undertaken with RCTs, and there is existing guidance for writing proposals in related areas such as mixed methods research. In this chapter, existing guidance is introduced and built upon to offer comprehensive and detailed guidance for writing a proposal for qualitative research undertaken with an RCT. There are challenges to writing these proposals and these are discussed and potential solutions proposed.

7.1 Types of proposals

Research proposals are required for a range of purposes and the guidance reported in this chapter is relevant to all these. This chapter focuses on writing research proposals rather than completing application forms which are also necessary for submission to these bodies:

Grant proposals for funding agencies. Researchers need to write proposals to gain funding. Each funding body has a unique application form which needs to be completed alongside an accompanying research plan or proposal. These application forms and proposals are then considered by members of the funding board, and by external reviewers prior to the funding board meeting.

Proposals for ethics committees/institutional review boards. Researchers need to seek ethics approval for any study involving human beings. Institutions and health organizations have their own boards or panels to assess ethics and their own unique application forms. A research proposal is required alongside the application form.

Proposals for PhDs. Graduate students often need to write detailed proposals for their PhDs, which are then reviewed by academic boards internal to their university. Sometimes students undertake qualitative research for their PhDs while an externally funded research team undertake the RCT. Alternatively, students may undertake the feasibility study for an RCT as their PhD, combining qualitative research and a pilot RCT. The guidance in this chapter is relevant to both of these scenarios.

Published protocols. It is standard practice to publish the protocol for an RCT so that reviewers can compare the planned and completed studies. It is becoming increasingly common to publish the protocol for the qualitative research or process evaluation undertaken alongside an RCT, either as part of the protocol for the RCT (e.g., Smith et al., 2014; Thomas et al., 2014) or within a separate protocol (e.g., Ellard et al., 2011; Grant et al., 2012). These protocols are based on the original grant proposals but usually offer more detail because plans have progressed further.

7.2 Existing relevant guidance for writing proposals

There is a range of published guidance relevant to writing proposals for using qualitative research with RCTs:

Guidance for writing proposals for qualitative research with RCTs. Drabble et al. (2014) focus on the process of writing the qualitative research component of a mixed methods evaluation. They undertook a documentary analysis on 32 successfully funded proposals, identifying good practice and key missing information. They offer a short set of recommended items for inclusion in proposals.

Guidance for undertaking qualitative research in feasibility studies for RCTs. O'Cathain et al. (2015) offer guidance on undertaking qualitative research at the feasibility phase of an RCT. This guidance considers the spectrum of planning, undertaking, and reporting the qualitative research but much of it is relevant to writing a proposal. The guidance is reported in Chapter 4 Table 4.1.

Designing a process evaluation. Moore et al. (2015) offer recommendations for designing a process evaluation which includes quantitative and qualitative methods. This guidance considers the whole spectrum of planning, undertaking and reporting a process evaluation but much of it is relevant to writing a proposal.

Writing a proposal for mixed methods studies in health. Curry and Nunez-Smith (2015) devote a chapter of their book about mixed methods in health to how to select a funder, communicate with funders, develop a realistic timeline for a mixed methods study, and write a research proposal. They offer details of three real world grant applications—large, small and career development grants—to the US funder the National Institutes of Health. They also include tips based on interviews with members of funding boards and successful applicants.

Writing a mixed methods application for the US National Institutes for Health. Creswell et al. (2011) describe best practices for writing mixed methods proposals for a range of grant types to the US National Institutes of Health Research (https://obssr.od.nih.gov/training/mixed-methods-research/). The guidance follows the sections of the application forms, offering detail for the content of each section and references researchers can use.

Writing a proposal for a mixed methods study. Creswell (2002) summarizes the key content required for a mixed methods research proposal in a chapter in this book. Creswell and Plano Clark's book (2007) is essentially guidance for designing a mixed methods study.

Writing a proposal for qualitative research. Many universities publish guidance on their websites for students planning to write proposals for undertaking qualitative research to gain an academic qualification. Some researchers have reflected on writing qualitative research proposals. For example, Connelly and Yoder (2000) identify a number of common failings in qualitative research proposals such as a lack of rationale for using qualitative research and inadequate explanation of methods. Sandelowski and Barroso (2003) draw attention to how writing a proposal is as much of an art as a science.

Writing a research proposal. Books are available which detail how to write a research proposal for research generally (e.g., Punch 2016).

7.3 Guidance for the content of a research proposal

Guidance for writing a research proposal for the qualitative component of a mixed methods evaluation is offered in Table 7.1. The foundation of this guidance is Drabble et al. (2014), expanded using the range of wider guidance detailed in Section 7.2. The strength of Drabble et al's guidance is that it is short and can be used when space is limited, for example when writing a grant proposal. The strength of the expanded guidance in Table 7.1 is that it can be used when researchers need to plan their study in detail.

7.4 Challenges and potential solutions

7.4.1 Not enough space on application forms

A number of scholars have found that the qualitative component in a mixed methods research proposal tends not to be described in detail (O'Cathain et al., 2008; Creswell et al., 2011; Curry and Nunez-Smith, 2015). For example, O'Cathain et al. (2008) assessed 45 proposals of a key UK funding body, including some combining RCTs and qualitative research, and found that 42% of qualitative components lacked sufficient detail compared with 18% of quantitative components. A more recent study of 32 proposals of qualitative research and RCTs registered on a trials database found that a quarter used a single paragraph or less to describe the qualitative research (Drabble et al., 2014). Key information was missing in a large minority of proposals, particularly about sample size, type of analysis, and non-personnel resources. There were even examples of a single sentence only to describe the qualitative research, which was then repeated in different parts of the proposal. This issue may no longer be relevant today as researchers and funders understand the importance of the qualitative research. However, this problem may persist today because of the value the lead investigator places on the qualitative research; space is a precious resource in a word limited research proposal and the preference may be to use this space for what is most valued—the RCT. The content of a research proposal can also be shaped by research communities' expectations in that they hold strong views about what information is essential when planning an RCT but are not clear about essential details for any associated qualitative research. Researchers experienced in combining qualitative research and RCTs have suggested that this issue could be addressed by structural change, with funding bodies changing application forms to offer explicit space for the qualitative research (O'Cathain et al., 2014b). Agency could also be a solution, with reviewers and panel members requesting sufficient detail if this is not given,

Table 7.1 Guidance for researchers writing proposals for the qualitative research undertaken with RCTs

Consistency across the proposal	Attention to the qualitative research throughout the proposal (and application form) is needed so that those assessing the proposal can see that the qualitative research is an integrated component of the whole evaluation
Literature review	Include references to relevant qualitative research for the patient group, type of intervention, or context in which the RCT will be undertaken. Show how the plan for the whole evaluation will attend to this learning and how the qualitative research will build on existing evidence
Rationale for the qualitative research	Describe the rationale for including the qualitative research by writing a statement addressing the ways in which the qualitative research will add value to generating evidence of effectiveness in conjunction with the RCT. See Chapter 1 for different rationales to select from
Aim	Describe the aims of the qualitative research. These should be based on the key uncertainties identified in the literature, key stakeholders and the research team. Link these aims to the RCT, for example, 'to explore patients' views of the intervention' rather than 'to explore patients' experiences'. See Chapter 3 for the range of contributions qualitative research can make to RCTs and Chapter 8 for examples of aims
Framework	Place the whole mixed methods intervention evaluation within one of the frameworks described in Chapter 2. There is no right framework; some research communities favour particular frameworks
Design	The qualitative research may be undertaken before, during or after the full RCT so describe its relationship with RCT. It may be undertaken alone or as part of a mixed methods process evaluation. It is not necessary to use a named design. Reference any relevant published guidance available for this design (see Chapter 2)
Paradigm	It is not common to describe paradigms in grant proposals (see Chapter 5). PhD students in some academic disciplines will be expected to describe the paradigm in which they are working and justify its selection. Students will need to seek information from supervisors about expectations concerning discussions of paradigms
Theory	Is there a theory that is relevant to the intervention or its implementation? If so, describe its relevance and how it will shape the qualitative research (see Chapter 6)
Methodological approaches and methods	The qualitative research may be undertaken within a methodology or approach such as ethnography or case studies. If so, describe justify and reference the approach. Description and referencing of common methods is not usually required in grant or ethics proposals but is required for PhD proposals (e.g., interviews, focus groups). Justification for the methods selected is useful, e.g. telephone interviews, focus groups, dyadic interviews (see Chapter 9)

(*continued*)

Table 7.1 Continued

Data collection	Provide a clear account of the proposed methods of data collection including the location and timing of data collection, and the skills and seniority of the person who will undertake data collection. Describe issues specific to the patient group, intervention or context e.g. the expertise of a researcher in working with people with learning disabilities in an RCT of obesity reduction in this group. See Chapter 9
Sampling	Describe the sample frame, sampling approach, and likely upper and lower range for the sample size. Where the sample frame is RCT participants, specify whether intervention, control or both will be included. Diversity of sample is important, particularly in the context of feasibility studies. See Chapter 9
Recruitment	Institutional Research Boards and Ethics Committees will want details about who will approach patients and how informed consent will be taken
Analysis	Describe and reference the proposed approach to analysis. A rationale for the approach to be taken can be included. Specify timing of analysis e.g. an intention to undertake analysis prior to the RCT outcomes being known. See Chapter 10
Integration with RCT	Outline plans for integrating the qualitative data or findings with the quantitative process evaluation data or the RCT results. See Chapter 11
Challenges	Describe any challenges specific to undertaking the qualitative research with this patient group, intervention or context, and how they will be addressed. For example, if interviews are to occur in a number of countries and languages, discuss how translation will be handled
Rigour	There are criteria for undertaking high quality qualitative research. These are paradigm dependent so some sets of criteria only will be relevant to the evaluation. There may be issues specific to using qualitative research with RCTs such as attention to the potential for the qualitative research to contaminate the RCT. If there is a risk of this, specify the actions to be taken to mitigate the risk. See Chapter 13
Ethical issues	There may be additional issues to attend to above and beyond a qualitative study. For example, is there risk of breach of confidentiality if qualitative findings are fed back to teams which include clinicians treating the interviewees? Will there be the potential to overburden participants who complete data collection for both the qualitative research and the RCT?
Patient and public involvement	Appreciate the difference between qualitative research and Patient and Public Involvement. Specify the role of Patient and Public Involvement members in the qualitative research as well as the RCT and whole evaluation (see Chapter 15)

(continued)

Table 7.1 Continued

Costs	Describe the full costs of the qualitative research and highlight any dedicated equipment, software, staff, and transcription needed. Interviewees may need to be paid for travel, their time or to cover caring needs for the time they spend being interviewed
Leadership	Identify which of the co-applicants will take overall responsibility for the qualitative research and describe their role in the design, data collection, analysis and reporting of the study
Team	Describe the expertise of the qualitative researchers who will undertake the data collection, analysis and reporting. This expertise can relate to qualitative research generally or be specific to the patient group, intervention or context of the RCT. Attention could be given to how these team members will work with the wider team in terms of integrated or separate working (see Chapter 14)
Relationship with wider stakeholders	Think about the benefits and risks of having working relationships with intervention developers and those implementing the intervention. The approach can then be documented in the proposal (see Chapter 15)
RCT infrastructure	The qualitative research may engage with traditional RCT infrastructure, for example with formal submissions to the Trial Steering Group and use of Standard Operating Procedures (See Chapter 15).
Timetable	It can be time consuming to undertake data collection and analysis in qualitative research. Specify the timing so reviewers can judge if enough time has been allowed
Environment	Describe how the academic environment of the institutions involved in the evaluation is conducive to mixed methods research, for example if the Clinical Trials Unit has a history of working with qualitative research (see Chapter 15)

Reproduced with courtesy of the author.

lead investigators allocating sufficient space for the qualitative research when writing a proposal, and qualitative researchers pushing for enough space to describe their proposed work.

It is also worth considering which issues are essential to describe within different types of proposals. For example, recruitment details are essential for an ethics or PhD proposal but desirable for a grant proposal unless recruitment of a specific patient is seen as challenging.

7.4.2 Funders' and reviewers' lack the expertise

In the past, qualitative research with RCTs may have been dismissed, ignored, or misunderstood because members of funding bodies and ethics panels have been largely or totally quantitative researchers with little understanding of the value of qualitative research. It is now much more common to have qualitative, mixed methods researchers and Patient and Public Involvement representatives on funding boards and ethics committees so there should be the right expertise to judge the qualitative research (O'Cathain et al., 2014b). In addition, funding bodies are likely to seek the views of reviewers with qualitative research expertise where there are qualitative components in a grant proposal. It is also more likely now that quantitative researchers understand the complexity of interventions and so are extremely supportive of using qualitative research with RCTs. It is important that lead investigators ensure that space is allocated to the qualitative research and that details are given to allow reviewers to make judgements about the utility and quality of the proposed research.

7.4.3 Not enough money

Qualitative research costs money to undertake, especially if it is to be undertaken to a high standard. Studies where researchers reported there were senior qualitative researchers as applicants with enough of their time funded to ensure good-quality research was undertaken and qualitative researchers to undertake the research rather than trial managers doing it alongside running the RCT, with enough time allocated to allow for an in-depth qualitative analysis, were described as taking the qualitative findings seriously and maximizing the potential of the qualitative research (O'Cathain et al., 2014a). Researchers can be concerned that funders will not be willing to spend a lot of money on the qualitative research and may cut resources to make it more fundable (O'Cathain et al., 2014a). Attention to value for money is important (see Chapter 1) and researchers can address this issue by clearly communicating why the qualitative research is important (the rationale) and the contribution it will make. Researchers themselves can put costs and planned contributions side by side and assess whether they consider the qualitative research to be good value for money. Then they can reduce costs or make a clear case for the original funding so that reviewers might also draw the same conclusions.

7.5 Key points

- Detailed guidance for writing a research proposal is given in Table 7.1.
- This guidance is relevant to different types of proposals including those for funding, for ethics approval, for research degree approval, and published protocols.

- Although researchers face some structural challenges, the context is becoming favourable to writing and reviewing proposals for qualitative research with RCTs.
- Researchers can take action themselves to address the challenges faced.

7.6 Questions to help you think about your study

- How much space have you allocated in the proposal to describe the qualitative research?
- If you are not the lead investigator, what generic parts of the proposal do you have to write or contribute to writing so that the proposal is consistent?
- If space is limited, what will convince the reviewers and funders that you intend to undertake a useful piece of qualitative research, it is worth the money, and you know what you are doing?

Further reading

Drabble, S.J., O'Cathain, A., Thomas, K.J., Rudolph, A., Hewison, J., 2014. Describing qualitative research undertaken with randomised controlled trials in grant proposals: a documentary analysis. *BMC Medical Research Methodology*. Volume 14, P. 24.

Chapter 8

Selecting research questions

Overview

Read this chapter to learn about

- Factors that shape the selection of research questions
- Types of research questions in proposals and published protocols
- Challenges in selecting questions and potential solutions

Qualitative research can make a wide range of contributions to the generation of evidence of effectiveness (see Chapter 3). Researchers do not necessarily set out with the intention to address these issues. That is, researchers can start with a broader set of research questions, and then specific issues can emerge during the qualitative analysis that are considered to be important enough to become the focus of journal articles. In this chapter consideration is given to the research question, or set of research questions, articulated in the proposal or published protocol. Issues addressed in the chapter include the factors shaping the selection of research questions, examples of research questions used in proposals and publications, and challenges faced when selecting research questions.

8.1 Factors affecting the selection of research questions

A wide range of factors can affect the selection of research questions for the qualitative research.

8.1.1 Uncertainty

The main driver of selection of research questions should be uncertainty. For full RCTs there is likely to be future uncertainty about why the intervention was effective or not. This future uncertainty can be addressed at the planning stage of the evaluation by organizing to undertake qualitative research alongside the full RCT. For complex interventions, the qualitative research can focus on understanding the three functions of a process evaluation (Moore et al., 2015): mechanisms of impact of the intervention, how the intervention was implemented, and the contribution of the context in which the intervention and RCT operated. In feasibility studies for RCTs there may be uncertainty about how health practitioners will actually deliver the intervention (feasibility), or how patients will engage with the intervention (acceptability), or whether sufficient numbers can be recruited for the full RCT.

8.1.2 **Concerns**

As well as uncertainty, there can be significant concerns or scepticism within the research team or from external stakeholders such as funding bodies about the intervention, the outcomes measured or the ability to recruit for a full RCT. Although researchers and funders are always concerned about RCT recruitment, the concern may be significantly greater for a particular RCT because of

- the intervention (it may be at risk of being viewed negatively by the target patient group),
- the target patient group (they may be a transient population),
- who will recruit (perhaps the recruitment process is complicated long and the proposed practitioner has a heavy workload), or
- the context in which the RCT is undertaken (perhaps recruitment will take place in a dispersed rural community).

A feasibility study for the full RCT can be undertaken to show that these concerns were supported and problems were fixable, or that the problems did not occur in practice.

8.1.3 **Research evidence**

Research evidence may generate concerns and thereby contribute to the identification of a research question. For example, a literature search of previous RCTs with a patient group may identify that these RCTs have always failed to meet recruitment targets. Alternatively, a literature review may reduce uncertainty if researchers have already identified solutions to address concerns held by the research team. Additionally, searching for previous relevant qualitative research can direct the team to more specific research questions. For example, previous qualitative research may have identified that problems with recruitment for particular RCTs lie with recruiters rather than patients and the research question can then focus on how recruiters implement recruitment procedures.

8.1.4 Level of innovation

Some evaluations may focus on very different types of interventions from those operating in usual care or evaluated previously. Or the delivery of an intervention may be innovative. Previous research may not be suitably relevant and this increases the amount of uncertainty held by the research team. Even where similar interventions have been evaluated in similar contexts, there will still be uncertainty about whether this particular complex intervention used in this specific context will be implemented as planned. That is, qualitative research may be necessary even where there is a large amount of relevant research evidence about previous interventions.

8.1.5 Paradigms and theories

The paradigm may shape the questions asked. For example, an implementation science paradigm may focus attention on research questions related to how best to implement the intervention in the real world. The intervention or its implementation may be based on or informed by a theory or theoretical framework. Components of this theory will certainly inform the data collection and topic guides, and may also inform the research questions. See Chapters 5 and 6.

8.1.6 Type of RCT

Researchers undertaking cluster RCTs may expect differences in effect sizes between the clusters, generating a research question of why outcomes differed between clusters. Qualitative research alongside N of 1 trials may focus on why differences in outcomes occurred between individuals. See Chapter 4.

8.1.7 The rationale for undertaking the qualitative research and the RCT

The rationales for using qualitative research with RCTs were addressed in Chapter 1. These rationales can be shaped by paradigms or uncertainties held by the research team, and these in turn will affect the research questions (see Box 8.1). When Drabble et al. (2014) studied 32 successful grant proposals, they found that where the rationale was mentioned, it concerned optimization of implementation of intervention in the real world, improving the RCT conduct, interpreting the RCT results, and generating theories about the intervention.

8.2 Types of questions

In his book directed at helping undergraduate students undertake research, Bryman states that research questions should not be too broad (Bryman, 2012). Drabble et al. (2014) found that many of the stated aims in 32 grant proposals

Box 8.1 Example of how the rationale for the qualitative research shapes the research questions

Wiart and colleagues' (2016) study protocol for a 'mixed methods RCT' of an intervention to improve the gait of children with cerebral palsy was introduced in Box 2.1 in Chapter 2. The objectives of the concurrent qualitative component were three-fold: to identify the child and parent experiences of the interventions, the outcomes important to families, and the factors influencing participation in the RCT. The researchers offered a number of justifications for these three objectives. A driving rationale of the researchers appeared to be to understand the implications of the intervention for clinical practice in the real world. They also had the rationale of explaining the RCT results but this appeared to be secondary to the rationale of implementation in clinical practice. The researchers were interested in how to ensure children and parents were engaged and motivated with their therapy (shaped objective 1), to understand the goals parents have in their therapy (shaped objective 2), and how strong parental preferences for different types of therapy might affect use of the therapy in practice as well as cause recruitment difficulties in the RCT.

Source: data from Wiart, L., et al. 'Evaluation of the effectiveness of robotic gait training and gait-focused physical therapy programs for children and youth with cerebral palsy: a mixed methods RCT'. *BMC Neurology*, **16**, 86. doi: 10.1186/ s12883-016-0582-7. Copyright © Wiart et al. 2016

of studies combining qualitative research and RCTs were broad, for example 'to explore patients' views and experiences of the intervention'. They also identified more specific aims, for example 'to gain insights into reasons for lack of adherence to the intervention'. The strength of a broad research question is that it keeps the field of enquiry open and wide, helping to ensure that any important issues are identified. This is important because researchers may not be clear about which issues might derail the intervention when planning their evaluation. The strength of a narrow research question is that it shows that the researchers have thought about the aspects of the intervention or RCT about which there is more uncertainty. Creswell and Plano Clark (2007) suggest the best of both worlds when discussing research questions for mixed methods studies. They recommend having a broad question followed by a number of more narrowly focused questions. This may be a useful way of articulating the research questions for qualitative research with RCTs, in terms of having aims followed by a number of specific objectives. An example of this is given in Box 8.2. The key issue is that researchers give thought to how broad or narrow they wish their questions to

Box 8.2 Example of aims and objectives in a published protocol for a process evaluation

Jack and colleagues (2015) published a protocol for the process evaluation alongside an RCT of the family nurse partnership, an intervention of health professionals visiting the homes of disadvantaged mothers. The rationale for the RCT was that the intervention had been shown to be effective in the USA but not in the different context of Canada. Therefore, context was important to the research team. The process evaluation was a mixed methods study, with some research questions addressed by quantitative research and others by qualitative research. The primary aims of the process evaluation were similar to those set out by process evaluation guidance: to describe stakeholders' perceptions of the intervention, to assess delivery fidelity, to describe implementation and to describe contextual factors that might explain differences in outcomes in the five geographical areas participating in the RCT. The team expected that there might be differences in outcomes between the five areas and so established an aim to explore implementation and context between these five areas. The team then articulated eight detailed objectives to address these aims. Quantitative research was planned to address fidelity. Qualitative interviews and focus groups were planned with all 71 practitioners delivering the intervention and with five to 15 managers annually. The objectives addressed by this qualitative data collection focused on specific issues important to the research team undertaking the evaluation in Canada, such as education and training for the workforce, experiences of delivering the intervention to specific groups, and experience of delivering it within non-urban areas.

Source: data from Jack, S.M., et al. and BCHCP Process Evaluation Research Team. (2015) British Columbia Healthy Connections Project process evaluation: a mixed methods protocol to describe the implementation and delivery of the Nurse-Family Partnership in Canada. *BMC Nursing*, Issue 14, p. 47. Copyright © Jack et al. 2015.

be rather than writing a broad research question because they have not thought through the issues they are keen to know more about within their specific study.

8.3 Examples of research questions

Examples of broad and narrow research questions are shown in Table 8.1 within the 'aspects of an RCT' framework described in Chapter 2.

Table 8.1 Examples of research questions

Aspect of RCT	Broad	Narrow
Intervention	Is the intervention acceptability and feasibility? Is the intervention implemented as planned?	Why is compliance with the intervention poor? What are the key differences between the intervention and usual care? Can the workforce delver the intervention within their routine practice? How do practitioners deliver each of the key components of the intervention?
	What are the mechanisms of action of the intervention?	How do patients value each of the components of the intervention?
	How does context affect implementation and outcomes?	How does the organizational context in which the intervention is offered affect implementation? Does context vary in each RCT site in ways that might affect the outcomes achieved?
Conduct	Is recruitment as effective as possible?	Can recruitment rates be improved? How do preferences for the intervention affect recruitment? How should informed consent best be obtained? How can diversity of recruitment participants be maximized?
Outcomes	What outcomes are important to patients?	Are all important outcomes being measured in the full RCT? Do patients place different values on the different outcomes?
Measures	Are the proposed measures suitable for use in the RCT?	What is the content validity of the outcome measures for the target group?

Reproduced with courtesy of the author.

8.4 **Challenges and potential solutions**

8.4.1 **Addressing the numerous uncertainties**

In order to gain the most benefit from process evaluations, Linnan and Steckler (2002) suggest that researchers focus on the most salient processes to reduce the volume of data collected, particularly if cost is an issue. Researchers will have to prioritize research questions by selecting the most important questions for their study from the range of questions identified, taking the resources available to them into consideration. It is best to involve the full research team in this decision-making process, including those leading the RCT and the qualitative researchers. Sometimes researchers are concerned that funders will not fund large amounts of qualitative research and may limit the scope or resources requested for it (O'Cathain et al., 2014a). Justifying why qualitative research is necessary, and why the selected research questions are important, can help funders to make decisions about value for money.

8.4.2 Being in 'generic mode'

Researchers who have undertaken a number of qualitative components or process evaluations can fall victim to using the same generic paragraph for each study, including the same generic research questions. It may be appropriate to focus on the three functions of a process evaluation—mechanisms of impact, implementation and context—but the importance of aspects of these may differ by study. In the example described in Box 8.2, Jack et al. (2015) avoid this pitfall by specifying the types of contextual factors that they are interested in: individual, organizational, cultural, social, and geographic.

8.4.3 Multiple ways of stating the same research question

Because there a number of ways of stating a research question, researchers can use different language to essentially describe the same thing. Exploring practitioners' and patients' experiences of the intervention may be the same as exploring the implementation of the intervention or exploring the feasibility and acceptability of the intervention. There are also different levels of research question. These may confusing within research proposals because researchers can phrase and rephrase research questions in so many different ways. It might help if researchers articulate clearly

- the rationale for the qualitative research, that is, why it is included—e.g., to explore whether the full RCT is feasible because RCTs in this patient group have struggled to recruit;
- aim or overall purpose or intention of the qualitative research—e.g., to understand how to improve recruitment rates;
- objectives, that is the specific goals the research will achieve—e.g., to explore recruitment practice by exploring the views of recruiters and patients and observing recruitment sessions.

8.4.4 Planned vs. emergent questions

If the planned research questions are broad, more specific research questions may emerge at three points in the study:

During data collection for the qualitative study. Emergence of a potentially important issue during the early data collection in the qualitative research is to be expected and welcomed. It is part of a flexible and iterative approach to qualitative research and can direct further sampling and topic guide content. For example, at the beginning of the RCT a large proportion of people may only use the intervention once rather than the planned six times and the research team may be so concerned about this that they direct sampling to include these patients. Or early interviewees raise concerns about an aspect of the intervention that is the explored explicitly in later interviews.

During analysis of the qualitative data. For example, while addressing the generic research question about implementation of the intervention during interviews, practitioners may discuss the importance of an aspect of the intervention that has not previously been articulated in the logic model. The research team may view this as an important invisible aspect of the intervention that needs to be made visible. They may identify an emerging research question related to the description and content of the intervention which then guides further qualitative analysis and decisions about what to publish from the qualitative research (see Chapter 12).

During analysis of the RCT or quantitative process data. An unanticipated finding from the quantitative research may identify a new research question that needs to be explored within the qualitative research. Given that the process data should be analysed prior to the RCT outcomes being known (Oakley et al., 2006), any unanticipated findings identified by the RCT will occur when the qualitative data collection is complete. Qualitative researchers can return to their data to explore these issues retrospectively without recourse to further data collection. Munro and Bloor (2010) discuss the challenges involved in doing this and the 'explanatory burden' it places on the process evaluation (p. 702). Qualitative researchers may need to take a cautious approach to reporting the findings from this if they perceive that they lack the data to offer a robust explanation of unanticipated RCT findings.

8.5 Key points

- Research questions can be shaped by key uncertainties, concerns held by external stakeholders, research evidence, theory, the type of RCT and the rationale for the study.
- Research questions can be broad or narrow. Each approach has its strengths. A combination of broad aims and more specific objectives can be helpful.
- Numerous potential research questions may have to be prioritized and reduced to a practical number.
- Research questions can also emerge over time from the qualitative or quantitative research.

8.6 Questions to help you think about your study

- What is the range of *potential* research questions?
- Which research questions are prioritized by the research team and why?
- Are there narrow questions specific to your study as well as broad research questions?

Further reading

Creswell, J.W., Plano-Clark, V.L. (2007). *Designing and Conducting Mixed Methods Research* (2nd edn). Thousand Oaks, CA: Sage Publications.

Chapter 9

Collecting data

Overview

Read this chapter to learn about

- The range of qualitative methods used with RCTs
- The range of people who participate in the qualitative research
- Approaches to sampling
- Sample size
- Timing of data collection
- Who collects the data

There are many issues to consider when collecting data in qualitative research with RCTs. In this chapter consideration is given to the range of methods that can be used, who to include in the data collection, how to identify people or places to include, how many people or places to include, when to undertake data collection, and who is best placed to undertake it.

9.1 Different methods of data collection

The aim of this section is to describe the range of qualitative methods researchers have used with RCTs, indicate what each method can offer in this context, and give examples of their use so researchers can consider which methods are best for their study. This section does not offer detail about how to undertake qualitative methods. There are many excellent books offering introductions to researchers new to qualitative research who want to learn about these methods (Mays and Pope, 2000; Silverman, 2013). Methods can be undertaken within a methodology or approach, and the section begins with a description of these.

9.1.1 Methodologies or approaches

Morgan-Trimmer and Wood (2016) explore the benefits of using ethnography in the context of RCTs. Ethnography, which largely uses qualitative methods, is characterized by long-term engagement of researchers in the field, use of participant or non-participant observation, and use of other methods such as unstructured interviews, documentary analysis, and the researcher's field notes. The focus is a particular social or cultural group, with attention paid to culture and context. Morgan-Trimmer and Wood (2016) identify its benefits as threefold when used with RCTs: producing valid data through observing behaviours and events in real-life settings, rather than only through accounts given in interviews; understanding data within social contexts (context is a key issue for complex interventions and the complex environments in which RCTs occur); and developing and building intervention theory. The downside is that, in its purest form, it is time consuming and therefore expensive. However, researchers can use ethnographical approaches or 'applied ethnography' where they may use observation and interviews but spend less time in the field than classic ethnography might require. Ethnography has been used successfully with RCTs. Examples include its use in preparation for an RCT of an HIV intervention in the US (Garcia et al., 2015), at the feasibility phase of an RCT to improve recruitment for RCTs (Donovan et al., 2002), and alongside cluster RCTs to explain why an intervention was not effective (Hoddinott et al., 2010; Stapleton et al., 2002).

Researchers undertaking qualitative research with RCTs have also drawn on a case study approach (Yin, 2003). In their study of breastfeeding, Hoddinott et al. (2010) used ethnographic interviews, focus groups, observation, and surveys to understand implementation of the intervention in the seven intervention clusters in a cluster RCT. They described this approach as 'embedded mixed methods case studies' because each cluster was analysed as a case and then multiple case study analysis undertaken to explain why the effectiveness of the intervention differed by cluster. Case studies could also be used in the context of N of 1 trials (see Chapter 4).

9.1.2 Range of methods

In a mapping review of 296 peer-reviewed journal articles published between 2008 and 2010 that reported qualitative research undertaken with RCTs, data were extracted on the methods used in a purposive sample of 104 of the articles (O'Cathain et al., 2014b). Researchers used individual interviews, focus groups, non-participant observation, and recordings of consultations (Table 9.1). The sample of extracted articles was purposive rather than probabilistic because there had been no intention to count the frequencies of occurrences of key issues. With this is mind, the data offer a crude indication of frequency of use of different methods. In this time period, it appears that interviews and focus groups were used most commonly, with little employment of non-participant

Table 9.1 Range of qualitative methods used with RCTs between 2008 and 2010

Method	Numbers of articles out of 104	What method offers	Example*
Interviews (67 face to face semi-structured or depth, 9 telephone and 7 longitudinal/repeated)	83	Interviews were commonly used with professionals delivering the intervention and RCT participants. They offered depth of information on perceptions of individuals engaged with the intervention or the RCT	Romo et al. (2009), as part of an RCT in Spain of hospital-based heroin prescription compared with methadone prescription for long-term socially excluded opiate addicts, undertook in-depth semi-structured interviews with 21 patients receiving the intervention and paired family members. The aim of the qualitative research was to explore patients' and their relatives' experiences of the intervention as delivered within the trial
Focus groups	32	Focus groups were commonly used with professionals delivering the intervention and with RCT participants. They generated breath of information through interaction between participants' perceptions of the intervention or RCT	Pope et al. (2010), as part of a cluster RCT in South Africa of provider-initiated HIV counselling and testing of tuberculosis patients, undertook focus groups involving 18 trial intervention providers after the trial results were known. The aim was to explore the structural and personal factors that reduced the acceptability or feasibility of the intervention delivery by the clinic nurses
Non-participant observation	19	Researchers observed intervention delivery. This could identify differences between the planned intervention and the intervention in practice	Hoddinott et al. (2010), as part of a cluster RCT in the UK of community breastfeeding support groups to increase breastfeeding rates, undertook 64 ethnographic in-depth interviews, 13 focus groups, and 17 observations to produce a locality case study for each of 7 intervention clusters

(*continued*)

Table 9.1 Continued

Method	**Numbers of articles out of 104**	**What method offers**	**Example***
Audio recordings of consultations	3	If a key part of an intervention involved consultations between a service provider and a patient, recordings of these were used to describe the intervention in detail, understand fidelity and identify differences between the planned intervention and the intervention in practice	McQueen et al. (2009), as part of a RCT in the USA of a tailored interactive intervention compared with use of a generic website to increase colorectal cancer screening in primary care, audio-taped consultations involving 76 patients and 8 physicians, all of whom were participating in the RCT. The aim of the qualitative research was to explore the content and process of physician–patient discussions about screening during a visit to the physician
Diaries	3	In a small number of studies practitioners *delivering the intervention and RCT* participants kept reflective diaries. Sometimes these diaries were part of the intervention but were used also as part of the research, offering perceptions of the intervention	White and Winstanley (2009), as part of a RCT *in Australia of the benefits of introducing clinical* supervision for mental health nurses, collected diary data from 22 intervention recipients. The aim of the qualitative research was to explore the beliefs of those delivering the intervention about the acceptability of clinical supervision within the prevailing managerial culture
Other, e.g. documents, workshops	5	Documentary analysis was undertaken as part of a wider ethnography, or workshops as part of community based participatory research	

observation or analysis of audio-recorded consultations, diaries, or documents. One-off face-to-face interviews were the most common type of interview, with little use of longitudinal data collection. It is possible that some methods were used in practice but not reported in peer-reviewed journal articles. It is also possible that some of these methods are used more now.

9.1.3 Combinations of methods

Researchers often used methods in combination. Two common combinations were non-participant observation with interviews, sometimes undertaken within an ethnographic study, and interviews with focus groups. Sometimes the published articles focused on the findings of one method only, even where different methods had been used together in a wider qualitative study, and sometimes articles reported findings from all of the methods together in a single article.

9.1.4 Selecting methods

Selection of methods will depend on the research questions important within the qualitative study (see Chapter 8), the type of intervention, the setting in which the RCT is being undertaken, and the resources available. It may also depend on the expertise of the qualitative researchers designing the study but it is important that researchers do not let this limit selection of the most appropriate set of methods; researchers can always seek training in different methods.

It is easy to play safe within a research community and select the methods reported commonly in publications. It may be that perceptions of key individuals, and therefore interviews and focus groups, are the most useful source of data for a study, which is why they appear to be so commonly used. However, it may also be that researchers use these methods because they are familiar with them or learn that they are acceptable for use in this context. Hopefully by seeing the range of methods used by researchers in Table 9.1, and examples of their use, qualitative researchers can think about the combination of methods most suited to their study.

Some qualitative research undertaken with RCTs lends itself to non-participant observation and others to audio-recording. Where the whole intervention or a key part of it is offered in a single consultation or series of consultations, audio-recordings may offer a time-efficient way of observing the content of the intervention, how it is delivered in practice and how participants react to it. These recordings can be submitted to structured analysis to test the fidelity of the intervention delivery. They are also a source of rich data for in-depth qualitative analysis about the way patient react to the intervention (See Box 9.1). An added value of recordings is that they can be listened to by the

Box 9.1 Example of using qualitative analysis of audio-recordings of consultations

Schumacher and colleagues (2005) describe the qualitative research undertaken alongside an RCT of a cancer pain management intervention offering education, coaching, and support. Audio-recordings of intervention sessions were undertaken to assess fidelity but the research team realized that they contained rich data on how the intervention was operating. They applied for further funding to transcribe the recordings verbatim and analyse them in detail, and obtained further informed consent to do so. There were over 200 participants in the RCT so they selected a purposive sample for this qualitative component. The dataset was large so they identified three foci for in-depth analysis of the recordings. The study helped researchers to describe the coaching component of the intervention with more precision and understand why the intervention did not work for some patients. The intervention was refined based on this analysis.

Source: data from Schumacher, K.L., et al. (2005) Qualitative research contribution to a randomized clinical trial. *Research in Nursing and Health*, Volume 28, Issue 3, pp. 268–280. Copyright © 2005 Wiley Periodicals.

wider research team to engage the whole team in detailed understanding of the intervention content and delivery in practice.

9.2 Research participants

Who to include in data collection will depend on the research questions important for the qualitative study, the intervention, the context in which the RCT is being undertaken, and the resources available. A wide range of potential participants could be important within a study (Table 9.2). In the mapping review of 296 published articles reported in Section 9.1, when the aim of the qualitative research was to explore recruitment practices for the RCT, it was common to collect data from staff recruiting for the RCT and participants being recruited, including those who declined to participate in the RCT. When the aim was to explore feasibility, acceptability, and implementation of the intervention it was common to include staff delivering the intervention and patients receiving the intervention. An example of an interview study of patients receiving the intervention in an RCT is detailed in Figure 9.1; these interviews are reported separately from interviews with intervention

Table 9.2 List of potential participants in qualitative research

RCT participants	Practitioners	Wider stakeholders
Users of the intervention	Staff delivering the intervention	Staff in the wider organization in which the intervention is delivered
Participants in the control arm	Staff involved in usual care	Staff in organizations affected by the intervention
Those approached for recruitment to the RCT	Staff recruiting RCT participants	Policy makers
Participants who have stopped using the intervention Potential intervention users (feasibility phase) Family members caring for patients	Potential interventionists (in the feasibility phase)	

Reproduced with courtesy of the author.

providers which were published elsewhere. Further potential participants are staff and patients who are expected to give or receive the intervention in the RCT, who can be interviewed prior to the RCT to help to optimize the intervention prior to evaluation. Sometimes wider stakeholders can be included in data collection, for example, staff in the organization in which the intervention was delivered but who were not directly involved in delivery, or significant people in the lives of RCT participants such as parents of children or carers of frail elderly people.

It is usual to include practitioners and patients involved in delivery and receipt of the intervention in data collection. It may be helpful to justify why it is important to include other groups. For example, Wiart et al. (2016) considered the potential for the goals of the therapy being evaluated to differ for parents and children so planned to collect qualitative data on both groups.

Two groups worth further consideration for participation in qualitative research are participants in the control arm of RCTs and participants who cease to use the intervention.

9.2.1 Controls

Including participants from the control arm of the RCT was not common in the mapping review reported in Section 9.1 (O'Cathain et al., 2014b). Only seven of the 104 articles undergoing detailed data extraction reported inclusion of this group. Qualitative research can help to understand what treatments

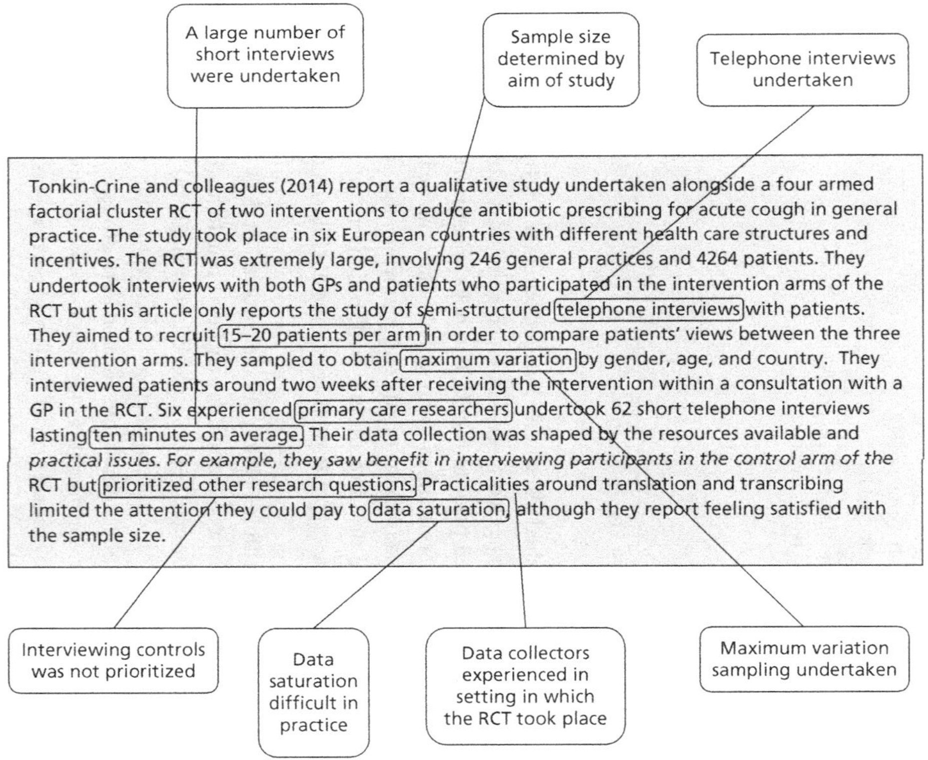

Figure 9.1 Example of data collection in a telephone interview study alongside a factorial cluster RCT

Source: data from Tonkin-Crine, S., et al. GRACE INTRO team. (2014). Exploring patients' views of primary care consultations with contrasting interventions for acute cough: a six-country European qualitative study. *Primary Care Respiratory Medicine*, Issue 24, Article number 14026, doi:10.1038/npjpcrm.2014.26. Open access.

participants in the control arm of an RCT are receiving in practice. It is worth considering the inclusion of this group in the qualitative research if there is little knowledge of what constitutes usual care (or active control) in practice. This is important because the choice of comparator for an RCT can affect the results of that RCT. If the proposed intervention is too similar to usual care then an expensive RCT may be a waste of money because the result is likely to be null. If usual care differs in different clusters of an RCT or even different recruitment sites in an individual-level multisite RCT then this may account for the different performance of the intervention in different contexts. The RCT may even change the provision of usual care within the RCT (McCambridge et al., 2014), and understanding this can affect interpretation of the RCT results and their proposed transferability to other settings.

Consideration of controls may be most useful at the feasibility phase in preparation for the full RCT so that action can be taken in terms of enhancing the intervention prior to use in the full trial (O'Cathain et al., 2015), or establishing ways of quantitative measurement of the content of usual care in the full RCT. Understanding usual care is also important during the full RCT because it represents a key feature of the context in which the new intervention will be implemented. Where a new intervention represents a fundamental change from usual practice, one would perhaps expect to encounter greater challenges to implementation, and practitioners would need to pay more attention to the resources and structures required to achieve change compared to where the intervention represents a more incremental change. Researchers can use qualitative research to explore usual care so that the intervention can be successfully integrated within it (Garcia et al., 2015).

Including participants from the control arm in the qualitative research may be viewed as useful but not a priority in the context of limited resources (see Figure 9.1).

9.2.2 **People who stop using the intervention early**

When using qualitative research to explore recruitment for an RCT, those who choose not to participate in the RCT are often interviewed as well as those who agree. People who stop using the intervention early are also a useful group to interview, especially when expected or actual drop-out rates are high. Researchers may face some resistance to this by ethics committee members concerned about the potential for harassing people. Experience in the Healthlines Study was that RCT participants who had stopped using the intervention for depression were happy to explain why they had done so in an interview and that this was extremely helpful in understanding patient engagement with the intervention overall (O'Cathain et al., 2016).

9.3 Sampling

9.3.1 Types of sampling

It is rarely possible to interview all the RCT participants receiving the intervention and sampling is likely to be required. Purposive sampling, and maximum variation sampling in particular, is commonly used in qualitative research with RCTs. There may be particular types of patients that are important to include in the qualitative research, for example, different genders because of expectations that men and women will react differently to the intervention. Diversity of characteristics is likely to be important for the qualitative research, particularly at the feasibility phase, when identification of negative views can help to enhance the intervention or RCT conduct for the full evaluation (O'Cathain et al., 2015). Maximum variation in terms of sex, age, and country was used in the example in Figure 9.1, presumably because the researchers believed that perceptions of the intervention might depend on these characteristics.

It is sometimes possible to interview all practitioners delivering the intervention, but in large RCTs it may be possible to interview only some of these. Researchers may have to think about the use of surveys in combination with the qualitative research if they wish to understand the perceptions of all the interventionists. Audrey et al. (2006) chose this approach when dealing with 30 intervention schools participating in a cluster RCT of a peer support intervention to reduce smoking in school children. They used questionnaires across the whole 30 schools and focused their in-depth process evaluation in four schools.

The type of RCT can influence sampling in the qualitative research. Cluster trials offer particular challenges for sampling because sampling may occur of clusters and then of individuals within clusters. Researchers may wish to undertake qualitative research within all the clusters. This can be extremely helpful in terms of understanding why different clusters appear to obtain different outcomes. This comprehensive approach to sampling is only feasible when there are small numbers of clusters (Hoddinott et al., 2010) and simply impossible in RCTs with large numbers of clusters (see example in Figure 9.1, where there are 246 clusters). Sampling different types of clusters may be the most feasible option. For example, Bosch et al. (2016) were planning a cluster RCT so in their preparatory work for this they undertook purposive sampling of staff for qualitative interviews from the range of types of organizations that would be clusters in the full RCT, that is, different sizes of organizations in different types of geographical areas.

Table 9.3 Pros and cons of different timing of the qualitative research

Timing of qualitative research	Benefits	Problems
Early days of intervention delivery or receipt	In a feasibility phase this can quickly identify problems that can be fixed In a full RCT this can identify problems which practitioners and patients will face in the real world	This may only identify 'teething problems' that the service delivering the intervention will fix regardless of feedback from qualitative research
When the intervention has 'bedded down' in the RCT	This gives a realistic view of intervention delivery when interventionists have gained some experience	In a feasibility study, the intervention may 'bed down' with large problems
Near the beginning of receiving the intervention	RCT participants can recall details about this important early stage of the intervention	No information about later stages of the intervention
At the end of receiving the intervention	RCT participants can comment on all the intervention	RCT participants may be unable to recall early stages of the intervention
After the primary outcome measurement	Eliminates concerns that any qualitative research can affect outcomes and thereby 'contaminate' the experiment	Contamination may not be a concern in reality and recall may be poor if the primary outcome measurement is at 12 months say
Different individuals at different times	The dataset has a mix of timings so includes a diverse range of views	Careful analysis is needed paying attention to the stage at which interviewees contributed data
Longitudinal data collection	Interviewees can recall details of recently used aspects of the intervention	Resources may not be available

Reproduced with courtesy of the author.

9.3.2 Selecting when to sample

Timing of data collection also needs careful consideration. The recruitment period for the RCT may occur over many months and researchers will have to consider when in this period the qualitative research is best undertaken—early in the RCT when there may be teething problems with the intervention or later when the intervention has bedded down. The intervention may be delivered to an individual over the course of a year and a decision will need to be made about whether to obtain early views of the intervention after a few months or wait until patients have received the full intervention. The pros and cons of different approaches are discussed in Table 9.3.

There is no right answer about when to sample participants. It is important to consider the gains and losses of different approaches for a particular study. For example, if practitioners and RCT participants are interviewed early in the provision trajectory of the intervention, then this can identify any significant 'teething problems' which could be fixed before the RCT continues. This is a useful approach to take in a feasibility study for a RCT where an iterative approach to data collection can result in optimization of the intervention or the RCT during the feasibility phase rather than waiting until the end of the feasibility study (O'Cathain et al., 2015; Donovan et al., 2016). Some timing decisions depend on the length of the intervention. The intervention from the patient perspective in the example in Figure 9.1 was one short consultation with a GP. Patients were interviewed around two weeks after the intervention. However in another study, the intervention lasted 12 months for each participant (Salisbury et al., 2016); the decision was made to interview participants at around six months, which was just after their primary outcome measurement (O'Cathain et al. 2016). This decision was made not because of concerns about contamination of the experiment (see Section 9.3.3), but because by then patients had experienced the majority of the intervention and this timing allowed for analysis and reporting before the end date of the funding.

9.3.3 Can the data collection damage the experiment?

A qualitative interview study of 18 researchers in the UK with experience of leading and working on studies combining qualitative and RCTs identified a concern among some that qualitative research could contaminate or damage the RCT by acting as an intervention (O'Cathain et al., 2014b). These researchers were concerned about the therapeutic effect of qualitative research, especially where the combination of interviews and observation were more intensive than the intervention under study. Being interviewed and observed could potentially help staff delivering an intervention to reflect on and improve their practice. Talking about their health or health care could prompt patients to take action to improve their health. If only patients in the intervention arm are interviewed then any therapeutic effect could damage the experiment.

Concerns about contamination can lead to triallists requiring that the qualitative data collection is undertaken after the primary outcome measurement in the RCT. This may not be necessary. In the context of an RCT where 300 patients receive an intervention over a year, interviewing 24 of these patients for one hour was considered to be unlikely to make a difference to the primary health outcome in the RCT (O'Cathain et al., 2016). However, in the context of an RCT where 30 patients receive an intervention, interviewing 24 of them or interviewing a smaller number three times and building up a relationship with them could possibly damage the experiment. Therefore the potential for contamination is something to consider in the context of a specific RCT rather than something that should be seen as a threat for all RCTs.

9.4 Sample size

9.4.1 Usual study sizes

The numbers of people to be interviewed, focus groups run, or sessions observed will depend on the phase of evaluation, the aims of the qualitative research, the size of the RCT, data saturation, and the resources available. The size of RCT is a significant consideration if it is small, thus limiting the numbers that can be included in the qualitative research. In the mapping review described in Section 9.1 (O'Cathain et al., 2014b), sample sizes of the 104 published qualitative studies varied enormously. Numbers of interviews with staff (usually but not always those delivering the intervention) varied between one and 155. Sometimes the numbers of staff delivering the intervention was small and all of them were included. Of the 29 journal articles in the mapping review that reported interviewing staff, 11 interviewed ten or fewer, and six interviewed over 20. Of the 53 articles reporting patient interviews, numbers varied between seven and 725, with a median of 24 interviews. Six studies interviewed 10 or less patients and seven were large qualitative studies of over 60 interviewees. The variety was just as large for numbers of focus groups, varying between one and 11 for staff (median two or three) and one and 219 for patients (median 13). Justification for a sample size is helpful. For example, Wiart et al. (2016) justify their sample based on previous qualitative research with their target group and normal samples sizes for this type of research.

9.4.2 Data saturation

Data saturation is a good justification for final sample sizes in studies. Grant proposals will need to give a range between which data saturation is expected, for example specifying that between 16 and 25 patients will be interviewed dependent on data saturation. It may not always be possible to continue interviewing until researchers consider that data saturation has been achieved. In the example in Figure 9.1 the researchers stated that the delay between interview, translation, and transcription made consideration of data saturation impractical.

9.4.3 Length of interview or observation

Although length of interview or observation is not always considered in the context of sample size, some interviews can be long (one to two hours) and others short. For example, in one study interviews with patients were often over an hour long while interviews with staff not directly involved in delivering the intervention were closer to 30 minutes (O'Cathain et al., 2016). In the example in Figure 9.1 the telephone interviews were very short: from four to 18 minutes, with a median of ten minutes. Longer interviews can yield rich data and offer insights into context, although this is not guaranteed.

9.4.4 Collecting too much data

There is a temptation to collect too much data in qualitative research and process evaluations (Munro and Bloor, 2010). That is why Linnen and Steckler (2002) recommend limiting the amount and type collected. Data collection is time consuming and can drain resources needed for analysis and reporting. Too much data can leave researchers overwhelmed and feeling unable to do justice to the data collected when analysing and reporting it.

9.5 Who collects the data

9.5.1 The trial manager or a qualitative researcher?

Undertaking qualitative research well requires expertise. This becomes most evident at the analysis and reporting stage of a study. This expertise can lie with a senior team member who supervises a junior member of the team to undertake the qualitative research. This junior member of staff can be the trial manager or a qualitative researcher employed exclusively to undertake the qualitative research. The first option may be selected due to limited resources but has problems including the challenges of dealing with competing demands, and the potential for emerging findings from qualitative research to affect the morale of the researcher managing the RCT (Simons, 2007).

9.5.2 Background of the qualitative researcher

Qualitative researchers can be grounded in different academic disciplines and sub-disciplines. It might be helpful to have a public health-trained researcher undertake the qualitative research for an RCT of a public health intervention, or a psychologist for a behaviour change intervention, because they understand the theories behind the interventions. Alternatively these researchers may have expertise in the condition under study (e.g., mental health), the body of interventions under study (e.g., telehealth), the setting in which the study takes place (e.g., primary care), the data collection methods (e.g., non-participant observation), a research approach (e.g., case studies), or in undertaking process evaluations alongside RCTs. It is unlikely that teams can find researchers who have expertise in all these issues; one key expertise may be sufficient.

9.6 Key points

- Think beyond interviews and focus groups and consider the range of qualitative methods available including non-participant observation.
- Think beyond interviews with interventionists and patients; consider the range of potential participants including controls who can illuminate the content of usual care.
- When interventions are delivered to individuals over a number of months, or participants for the RCT are recruited over a number of months, qualitative research can be undertaken in the early phase of intervention delivery or receipt or when all participants have received the intervention. Decisions about timing of data collection will depend on the RCT and the intervention.
- Sample sizes may vary depending on the size and type of the RCT as well as data saturation.
- Qualitative researchers exclusively delivering the qualitative research can come from a range of backgrounds.

9.7 Questions to help you think about your study

- What data collection methods do you want to use and why?
- Who will be your participants and why? Do you need to prioritize this list with your team?
- How many participants will you include in your study? What parameters affect this choice?
- When will you collect data: at the end of the intervention, after the primary outcome measurement, at different times during intervention delivery? What do you gain and lose at different time points?
- Who will undertake data collection? What are the advantages of different experiences and backgrounds for this researcher?

Further reading

Silverman, S.L. (2013). *Doing Qualitative Research*. Thousand Oaks, CA: Sage Publications.

Chapter 10

Analysing the qualitative data

Overview

Read this chapter to learn about

- The range of different approaches to analysis
- How researchers describe their analysis in grant proposals and journal articles
- Team involvement in analysis
- Challenges and potential solutions

Numerous books and journal articles have been written about how to analyse qualitative data. In this chapter the assumption has been made that readers know how to do this. The focus of the chapter is on how researchers have analysed qualitative data collected with RCTs. The chapter begins with a brief description of the range of approaches to analysis used in the context of qualitative research with RCTs, giving examples of how researchers describe their analysis. Consideration is then given to who can be involved in the analysis and the challenges researchers may face.

10.1 Range of approaches to analysis

Reading published protocols and journal articles of qualitative research undertaken with RCTs identifies that researchers use a wide range of approaches to analysis, and sometimes a combination of approaches within a single study. Examples of some commonly used approaches are given in Table 10.1. There is likely to be many more approaches that are perhaps used less commonly; for example, Donovan et al. (2016) used conversation analysis in their use of qualitative research to improve recruitment for specific RCTs. Researchers do not necessarily justify why they have used a specific approach when describing their analysis (Table 10.1). Drabble et al. (2014) analysed 32 successfully funded research proposals submitted to UK funding bodies. Where the analysis was described, the most frequently used approaches were constant comparison (19%), thematic analysis (19%), content analysis (13%), and framework analysis (9%).

Table 10.1 Range of approaches to analysis of qualitative data collected with RCTs

Approach	Useful references	Example	Justification given in example
Thematic Analysis	Braun and Clarke (2006)	Journal article: Masood et al. (2015)	Flexible, no prior theoretical framework
Framework	Ritchie and Spencer (1994) Ritchie and Lewis (2013)	Journal article: O'Cathain et al. (2016)	Not stated
Iterative approach using constant comparison (from grounded theory)	Strauss and Corbin (1990)	Journal article: Coupe et al. (2014). Their study is described in Box 6.3 Journal article: Lawton et al. (2015)	Not stated Not stated
Interpretative Phenomenological Analysis	Smith et al. (2009)	Journal article: Toye et al. (2016)	Not stated
Interpretive description for all aspects of the qualitative research	Thorne (2008)	Published protocol: Wiart et al. (2016), see Box 2.1 Published protocol: Jack et al. (2015), see Box 8.2	This approach is taken to the research, including the analysis. Any analysis approaches already described in this chapter are used if they allow immersion in the data before coding starts and theorizing of relationships between themes
Content analysis	Hsieh and Shannon (2005)	Journal article: Curran et al (2013), see Box 6.2	Not stated. However, the team coded data to the Theoretical Domains Framework
Combination of named approaches	Not applicable	Journal article: Tonkin-Crine et al. (2014) used both thematic and framework analysis, see Box 9.1 Journal article: Hoddinott et al. (2010) used grounded theory followed by framework, see Box 4.3	Thematic analysis allowed researchers to start in inductive mode to reduce the risk of being overly influenced by the team's initial ideas or the literature they had read. Framework analysis facilitated handling a large data set and comparisons between different intervention arms and different countries A grounded theory approach was undertaken for the analysis of qualitative data. Framework facilitated building a model of factors affecting implementation
Description of steps taken	Not applicable	Journal article: Bosch et al. (2016), see Box 6.1 Journal article: Garcia et al. (2015)	Not stated Not stated. However, does state that the analysis was shaped by the ethnographic approach taken to data collection, grounded in a social ecological framework

Reproduced with courtesy of the author.

10.2 Selecting an approach

There is no right or wrong approach to take when analysing qualitative research with RCTs. Selection can be guided by the overarching approach to the qualitative research (e.g., grounded theory, interpretive description) or the aim of the analysis (to understand how a known theory plays out in the data, or to take an inductive approach). Selection is also likely to be influenced by the experience of the qualitative researchers who may have used an approach in the past and have a thorough understanding of it, or by the credibility of an approach within the relevant research community in which the lead qualitative researcher works and intends to publish.

10.3 Key issues to describe in the analysis section of a journal article

The key issues to describe in the analysis section of a journal article are largely similar to that for any qualitative research. There is one extra issue to consider and this is identified in italics in this list:

- name of the approach
- key reference for the approach
- justification for using the approach (if space allows)
- what was analysed, e.g. verbatim transcripts of audio recordings, field notes, etc.
- key steps taken
- roles of each researcher involved, with a description of disciplinary background if relevant
- software used for data management if relevant,
- *the timing of the analysis in relation to the RCT analysis.*

When the qualitative research is undertaken alongside a full RCT, with a rationale of explaining the RCT results, it is important to analyse the qualitative data prior to the results of the RCT being known to reduce the potential for bias (Oakley et al., 2006; Moore et al., 2015). It is good practice to do this and state that it has been done in publications (e.g., see Box 10.1)

10.4 Team involvement in the analysis

The team responsible for the qualitative research or process evaluation will lead the qualitative analysis. Members of the team responsible for the RCT may be involved in discussions about the qualitative data and inform the formal

Box 10.1 Example of describing timing of the qualitative research

An educational programme was delivered in schools to improve exercise and healthy eating in children (Campbell et al., 2015). It showed no effect in a cluster RCT but there were beneficial effects with respect to reducing self-reported consumption of high-energy drinks, snacks, and screen-viewing time. An embedded mixed methods process evaluation was used alongside the RCT. This included observation of the intervention delivery, questionnaires completed by teachers, logs of intervention delivery and semi-structured interviews with teachers and parents. The process evalua tion concluded that the fidelity of intervention implementation was good but that teachers were not enthusiastic about the intervention which may have led to them not delivering the intervention as anticipated. When reporting their process evaluation findings in a peer-reviewed journal, the researchers were explicit that the analysts were blind to the outcome of the full RCT and submitted their final draft to the trial steering committee chair before seeing the RCT results. They then identify this as a key strength of their study because their conclusions about the implementation of the intervention were not influenced by knowing the size of effect of the intervention.

Source: Campbell, R., et al. 'Intervention fidelity in a school-based diet and physical activity intervention in the UK: data from Active for Life Year 5'. *International Journal of Behavioral Nutrition and Physical Activity*, Issue 12, p. 141. Copyright © Campbell et al. 2015.

analysis. Involvement of these wider team members is a good idea during a feasibility study for an RCT because they can take actions on improvements to the intervention and RCT conduct for the full RCT. During a full RCT the study leader will need to decide whether it is a help or hindrance for the RCT team to hear findings from the qualitative research prior to completion of the RCT because there is a possibility of this feedback damaging the experiment for some RCTs (Cooper et al., 2014).

10.5 Challenges faced and potential solutions

10.5.1 Too much data

There is a great temptation to collect large amounts of data because the RCT is large, the participants are diverse, or there are numerous research questions.

This becomes a real problem at the analysis stage where the strength of qualitative research lies in depth of analysis. The best solution to this problem is to resist temptation to undertake large amounts of data collection at the cost of analysing the data properly. Even in the context of ample resources, the volume of data generated by qualitative research can be challenging to analyse, and it may be necessary to focus on specific parts of the data only during the formal analysis.

10.5.2 Speed of analysis

In feasibility studies for RCTs, the wider team may want to hear the findings of the qualitative research early in the study so they can improve the intervention or RCT conduct during the feasibility study and undertake further qualitative research to identify further insights. This dynamic or iterative approach (see Section 4.3 in Chapter 4) can create a challenge for the qualitative researchers who will need to ensure that qualitative data collection starts promptly, transcriptions are undertaken quickly, and analysis is undertaken rapidly. It may be that confidence in findings will not be strong until the full analysis is complete so it is best if early findings are identified and communicated with due caution. Donovan et al. (2016) discuss their approach to rapid analysis in the context of using qualitative research to improve recruitment rates in specific RCTs.

10.5.3 Resources available

When UK researchers experienced in combining qualitative research and RCTs were interviewed, some qualitative researchers were concerned that their quantitative colleagues did not understand that formal analysis of qualitative data is time consuming (O'Cathain et al., 2014b). Study leaders need to be aware of this and ensure that qualitative researchers are employed long enough on the study to complete the qualitative analysis and publish it.

10.5.4 High expectations

There may be tension around expectations of the qualitative research and what can be delivered in practice. The wider team members may look to the qualitative research to answer a range of question with certainty, including questions which emerge during the RCT. Although the qualitative research may enrich understanding of the trial findings, this understanding 'will always be nuanced and qualified and rarely determinate' (Munro and Bloor, 2010, p. 710). An example of hard-to-meet expectations is given in (Box 10.2). A potential solution to this is a team discussion at the start of any mixed

Box 10.2 Example of high expectations of analysis of the qualitative data

Munro and Bloor (2010) discuss a process evaluation carried out alongside a feasibility study for a full RCT. The intervention was training influential school pupils as peer supporters to discuss smoking cigarettes or cannabis with peers to educate them about the dangers of smoking. The pilot cluster RCT had three arms: peer supporter training in cigarette smoking, peer supporter training in cigarette and cannabis smoking, and controls. One of the outcome measures was the intention to smoke cannabis in three months and at age 16. The researchers found that there was no evidence of an effect on intention to smoke cannabis in the intervention schools, but unexpectedly they found an increase in expectations among peer supporters that they would be smoking cannabis by the time they were 16. By the time this unexpected finding emerged, the process evaluation data collection was complete, and there were no resources for further data collection. Nonetheless, members of the wider team were keen to explain this unexpected finding. So the researchers had to analyse the data they had already collected. They did find a possible explanation but had little confidence in it because it had not been explored specifically in their data collection. The researchers argued that there is a danger of expecting too much from process evaluations.

Source: data from Munro, A., Bloor, M. (2015) 'Process evaluation: the new miracle ingredient in public health research?' *Qualitative Research*, Volume 10, Issue 6, pp. 699–713. Copyright © 2015, British Medical Journal Publishing Group.

methods evaluation to consider what the qualitative research can and cannot deliver.

10.5.5 Integrating with the quantitative research

Once the qualitative research is analysed, the study team may wish to integrate the qualitative and quantitative data or findings. The qualitative researchers will need to work closely with quantitative colleagues to do this (unless the same team is responsible for both the quantitative and qualitative research). There is limited guidance for researchers wishing to do this. Details of how to approach integration are given in Chapter 11.

10.6 Key points

- Researchers take a range of approaches to analysis of qualitative data including thematic analysis, framework analysis, constant comparison, and content analysis.
- There is no right approach. Selection depends on the approach taken to the qualitative research, the aim of the analysis and the expertise of the researcher.
- Describing the analysis is the same as in any other qualitative study with one exception: stating when the analysis was undertaken in relation to knowing the results of RCT if the qualitative research is undertaken to explain the results of RCT.
- Challenges include analysis of large data sets, analysing with tight timelines, and high expectations of the answers it can provide.

10.7 Questions to help you think about your study

- What are you aiming to do in your analysis?
- Is your usual approach to analysis appropriate for your current study?
- Do you need to seek training in analysis?
- When is it appropriate to feedback findings from your analysis to the wider team?
- When will the data be analysed and who will be involved in this?

Chapter 11

Integrating qualitative and quantitative data and findings

Overview

Read this chapter to learn how to integrate qualitative and quantitative data and findings:

- Where integration can occur within a study
- Integration techniques
- Integration between the qualitative research and the RCT outcomes
- Integration within a process evaluation

Integration is where one method influences in some way the objectives, sampling, data collection, analysis, or interpretation of the other methods within a mixed methods study, leading to 'the whole more than the sum of its parts' (Barbour, 1999). A key rationale for using qualitative research with an RCT is to influence interpretation of the RCT results (see Chapter 1), a rationale that requires integration of findings from the qualitative research and the RCT. Studies of qualitative research undertaken with RCTs have identified that publications often have no evidence of integration of findings (Lewin et al., 2009; O'Cathain et al., 2014b). That is, the promise of qualitative research helping to explain the RCT findings is simply not delivered in practice, or at least not in a way that is visible outside the original research team. The focus of this chapter is on the different places integration can occur within a mixed methods evaluation, the techniques that can facilitate integration, and examples of integration of qualitative and quantitative research in the context of RCTs.

11.1 Where integration can occur within mixed methods evaluation

There are different ways of thinking about integration in mixed methods research (Fetters et al., 2013). In evaluations, approaches to integration depend on whether an evaluation is viewed as

- a phased sequential mixed methods design, or
- a single phase mixed methods study with concurrent use of methods.

11.1.1 Integration in a phased sequential design

An evaluation can be viewed as a set of sequential phases. For complex interventions these phases have been identified in Chapter 2 as

- development,
- feasibility,
- evaluation, and
- implementation of the intervention (Craig et al., 2008).

In practice, these phases are likely to be undertaken iteratively rather than purely sequentially, that is with movement backwards and forwards between phases. However, there is an overarching sequential movement through these phases. It is common to use a sequential mixed methods design that starts with a feasibility study (e.g., qualitative research undertaken alongside a pilot RCT) and is followed by an evaluation (e.g., a process evaluation alongside a full RCT). The integration in this sequential design occurs at the end of the feasibility phase, where conclusions about the intervention and RCT procedures from the feasibility study are acted on to improve the intervention, RCT procedures, data collection, or analyses in the full RCT (see Figure 11.1). The qualitative research in the feasibility phase can act as

- a **'problem solver'** by identifying problems to be fixed prior to the evaluation phase (O'Cathain et al., 2014a). For example, qualitative research at the feasibility phase of an RCT resulted in the use of a different outcome measure in the full RCT (Farquhar et al. 2010);
- or a **'hypothesis generator'** for testing in the full RCT. For example, in the feasibility phase researchers undertaking the qualitative research may conclude that different groups of patients appear to engage to different extents with the intervention and that this might affect the outcomes they achieve. This may lead to researchers leading the RCT ensuring that they collect data on these patient characteristics in the full RCT and generate a priori subgroup analyses for testing in the full RCT.

In a wider mixed methods research context these activities would be labelled as integration. In the context of qualitative research and RCTs, this is unlikely to be labelled as integration because the framing of the phases of an intervention study creates expectations that learning from the feasibility phase (both the qualitative and quantitative research) will impact the full RCT (quantitative

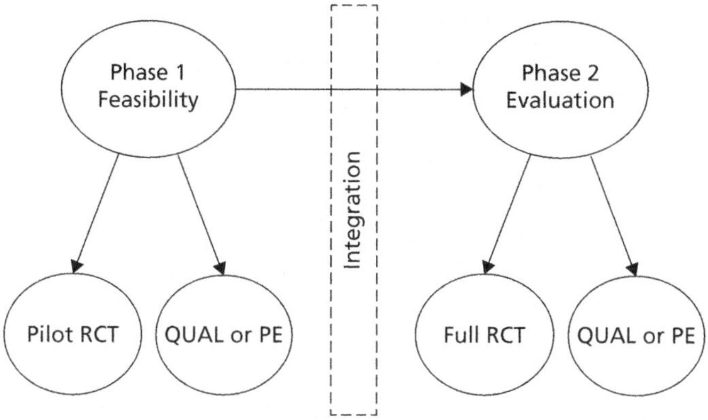

Figure 11.1 Integration in a sequential design
PE = mixed methods process evaluation QUAL = qualitative research
Reproduced courtesy of the author.

research). It is worth viewing this endeavour as integration because this may help researchers to be transparent about their actions prior to starting the full evaluation and consider whether any method or technique should be used for the integration. There will be cost and time implications associated with different outcomes of decisions, and uncertainty about whether changes will offer improvements in practice. Bugge et al. (2013) have developed a process for decision-making after pilot and feasibility RCTs to encourage the systematic identification and appraisal of problems, and associated potential solutions.

Feasibility phases for RCTs do not have to include a pilot RCT but where they do it is important not to treat the feasibility phase as if it were a mini version of the full evaluation (see Section 4.3 in Chapter 4). The feasibility phase is a learning phase where an iterative or dynamic approach to the qualitative data collection and analysis during the feasibility phase can influence RCT procedures in an ongoing way during the feasibility phase rather than waiting until the end of the feasibility phase (see Figure 11.2).

11.1.2 Integration in a single phase concurrent design

Integration is more complex for the concurrent use of qualitative and quantitative research within a single phase of the study, for example at the evaluation phase when there is a process evaluation and a full RCT, or the feasibility phase when qualitative research and a pilot RCT may be undertaken concurrently. One approach to integration is built into the design—the sample for the qualitative research is usually generated from the RCT participants and practitioners delivering the intervention. However, researchers must make extra efforts to

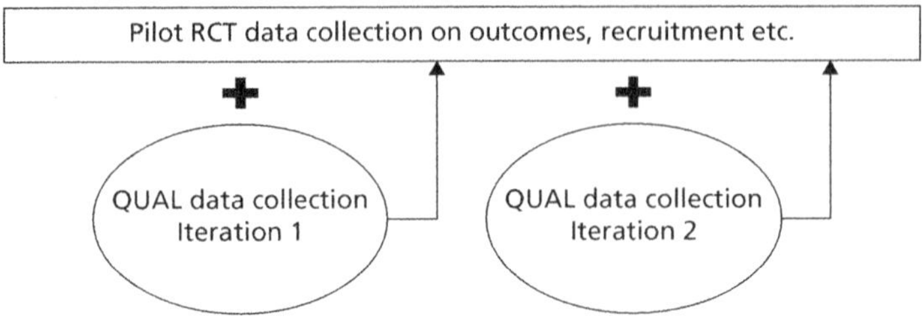

Figure 11.2 Integration within an iterative or dynamic approach to qualitative research during the feasibility phase
Reproduced courtesy of the author.

undertake further integration. Integration can occur in three places (see Figure 11.3):

- between the qualitative and quantitative research in a process evaluation (A),
- between the RCT outcomes and the qualitative research (B), and
- between the RCT outcomes and the process evaluation (C).

B and C are essentially the same. A distinction is made between them because Integration C may involve the integration of a large number of methods because process evaluations typically involve a number of quantitative (e.g., surveys, routine data) and qualitative methods (e.g., interviews, observation) which also need to be integrated with the RCT results.

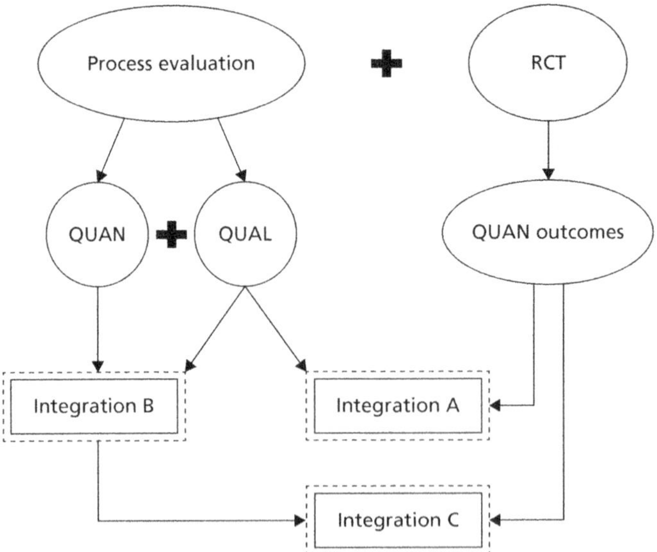

Figure 11.3 Integration in a single phase concurrent design
Reproduced courtesy of the author.

11.2 Integration techniques

Before considering different approaches to integration within mixed methods evaluations it is worth reviewing briefly three integration techniques relevant to mixed methods research more widely (O'Cathain et al., 2010). The first two techniques combine findings and the third technique combines data.

11.2.1 Integrating findings using an adapted triangulation protocol

Triangulation protocol was originally designed to integrate findings from different qualitative methods (Farmer et al., 2006). It has high utility for integrating findings from qualitative and quantitative methods (O'Cathain et al., 2010). Core steps can be used rather than following each step fully, resulting in the use of an adapted triangulation protocol. This involves analysing each dataset separately and identifying the findings from each dataset. These findings are then displayed side by side on the same page in 'meta-themes' within a matrix. Meta-themes cut across all data sets. Within a meta-theme, some findings may only occur in one dataset or may occur in a number of the data sets. The research team then compares and contrasts findings from different datasets within each meta-theme. They then consider where findings from each dataset are similar (agreement or convergence), complement each other (partial agreement or complementarity, for example where one explains, illuminates, or offers different information to other datasets), where findings contradict each other (dissonance or disagreement), or where findings do not occur in some of datasets but might have been expected to do so (silence). This offers a transparent and methodical approach to thinking about how the findings from different methods influence each other. After going through this process the research team will produce a set of meta-inferences from the whole mixed methods study (Teddlie and Tashakkori, 2009).

11.2.2 Working between findings and data sets using 'following a thread'

For this approach, each qualitative and quantitative dataset is analysed separately. A question may arise from one dataset which can be explored in the other dataset through further analysis of that dataset. The findings from this analysis may raise further questions that can then be explored in the first dataset. This 'thread' of thought and analysis (Moran-Ellis et al., 2006) may continue between datasets a number of times. In the context of qualitative research and RCTs the thread may be short and labelled as hypothesis generation and testing, where a hypothesis is generated from the qualitative research and tested in the

RCT dataset. The thread may be longer if the research team returns to the first dataset to refine the hypothesis for retesting in the RCT dataset.

11.2.3 Combining data using a mixed methods matrix

A unique aspect of mixed methods studies is that qualitative and quantitative data are available for the small number of RCT participants who have also participated in the qualitative research. For example, in depth interviews are undertaken with some participants in the intervention arm of an RCT, and outcome data from the RCT are also available for these individuals. These data can be displayed in a matrix, with RCT participants in rows ('cases') and different data on each case in columns ('variables'). Qualitative and quantitative data for a case can be compared and then patterns looked for across cases. This technique is used in qualitative analysis (Miles and Huberman, 1994) and transfers well to mixed methods studies.

11.3 Examples of different approaches to integration

There is a range of ways of integrating within studies involving qualitative research and RCTs. Eight approaches are described, and detailed examples are given for some of these.

11.3.1 Explaining the results of the RCT

A common rationale for undertaking qualitative research alongside an RCT is to explain the results of the RCT (integration A or C in Figure 11.3):

- **If an intervention has a large effect size** in the RCT it is important to understand how this was achieved so that practitioners in the real world can deliver the mechanisms of action of the intervention and achieve similar results. The large effect size may be dependent on context. The qualitative research can identify these mechanisms of action so they can be replicated post-RCT and identify important contextual issues so that practitioners in different contexts can consider the possibility of achieving similar outcomes.
- **If an intervention fails to show an effect** in the RCT then understanding whether the null result was due to poor mechanisms of action or failure to implement the intervention as planned can help direct future development of effective interventions.
- **If the effect size is small or modest** in the RCT, consideration can be given to whether and how the intervention could be improved to achieve a larger effect size. For example, a certain type of participant may not engage with

the intervention, leading to a hypothesis that focusing the intervention on a narrower target population might increase the effect size.

11.3.1.1 Explaining the primary outcome: triangulating conclusions

Some of the examples used throughout this book detail how qualitative research has been used to explain the results of an RCT. In Box 10.1 in Chapter 10, Campbell et al. (2015) use their process evaluation to explain why the RCT was null. They show how the teachers' lack of enthusiasm for the intervention may have resulted in poor delivery.

Where researchers use the qualitative research to explain the RCT results, it is not usual for researchers to explain how they did this. The first step is to analyse the qualitative data, or the qualitative and quantitative data within a mixed methods process evaluation. This is analysed prior to the RCT results being known (Moore et al., 2015; Oakley et al., 2006). Then the RCT data are analysed. Next, a journal article or report chapter is composed where the findings of the qualitative research are written up in a way that explains the RCT result. To do this, researchers need to triangulate the conclusions from the qualitative research and the RCT. That is, they consider whether the conclusions from each data set agree, partly agree or disagree and then consider why this is the case.

11.3.1.2 Agreement

The qualitative research may be fully aligned with the RCT result. In the example in Box 11.1 the qualitative research team wrote a draft report of their findings for the wider team prior to the RCT result being known. The qualitative team concluded at this stage that, given the strengths and weaknesses of the intervention, it would probably have some effect because interviewees described health improvements that they associated with the intervention, and the intervention was largely delivered as planned. However, the conclusion was also that significant problems with some aspects of implementation and context appeared to have had a detrimental effect on the intervention. This converged with the RCT result in that a modest effect was found. When writing the journal article from the qualitative research, the team reported this convergence of conclusions and then restructured the qualitative findings to tell the story succinctly of why this occurred (O'Cathain et al., 2016). There are three possible scenarios around convergence of conclusions which affect the focus of any publications:

- **The RCT shows a large effect size and the qualitative research concludes that the intervention was feasible and acceptable.** Here the journal article may focus on mechanisms of action and the contribution of context to the outcome, to allow practitioners to transfer this effect to their real world settings.

Box 11.1 Worked example of applying an adapted triangulation protocol to RCT and qualitative research findings

The RCT findings

An RCT of a telehealth intervention identified that it was not effective in terms of reducing overall risk for cardiovascular disease (CVD risk): adjusted odds ratio 1.3, 95% confidence interval 1.0 to 1.9 (Salisbury et al., 2016). There were reductions in the individual risk factors of high blood pressure and weight but not in the other risk factors of high cholesterol or smoking status. There were improvements in intermediate outcomes such as diet, physical activity, drug adherence, and satisfaction with access to care, treatment received, and care coordination. The more participants engaged with the intervention, the higher the effect size.

The qualitative research findings

An embedded qualitative research study was undertaken alongside the RCT: interviews with 21 practitioners delivering the intervention or working in health organizations offering health care to the RCT participants, and 12 participants receiving the intervention in the RCT (O'Cathain et al. 2016). The findings were that RCT participants in the intervention arm described improved outcomes which they attributed to the intervention. Key mechanisms of action were motivation to improve a specific risk factor, tailoring of the intervention to an individual's needs, and continuity of delivery by enthusiastic and motivated staff. These issues encouraged active engagement with the intervention by participants. Although the intervention was implemented largely as planned, there had been problems in the early part of the RCT: there were technical difficulties delivering the intervention, and a lack of continuity of intervention delivery tailored to individual patients' needs. Also, some patients joined the RCT for general health improvement or from altruism, rather than motivation to make lifestyle changes to address their specific risk factors. Engaging these unmotivated patients was seen as challenging by practitioners delivering the intervention. Finally, there was a lack of active engagement from primary care practitioners.

Adapted triangulation protocol

An adapted version of triangulation protocol was applied to the findings. A full triangulation protocol requires assessment of the quality of the research identifying each finding and this was not formally undertaken (Table 11.1). Also, thinking about complementarity rather than partial agreement can be more helpful in terms of identifying possible explanations.

Table 11.1 adapted triangulation protocol example

Theme	RCT	Qualitative	Convergence, complementarity, contradiction, silence
Change in overall CVD risk	Some improvement but uncertainty about this: OR=1.3 (1.0 to 1.9), p=0.08	Some interviewees talked positively about the intervention and how it addressed risk factors. They described the importance of continuity, enthusiasm, and tailoring by those delivering the intervention. However, there were problems in that some interviewees found the intervention of no use to them because they did not want to change or did not like the mechanistic approach to delivery. There were technical problems and delays at the beginning of the RCT. The expected collaboration with general practice was partial	Convergence in that both sets of data show evidence of improvement (recognizing that the RCT strength is measuring size of effect and the qualitative research is not designed to do this) Complementarity - findings from the qualitative research explain why some patients engaged with the intervention and others did not
Mean blood pressure	Reduced	Some patients discussed monitoring their blood pressure as part of the intervention, identifying high blood pressure and taking drugs or changing drug doses	Convergence

(continued)

Table 11.1 Continued

Theme	RCT	Qualitative	Convergence, complementarity, contradiction, silence
Mean weight and body mass index	Reduced	Some patients joined the RCT to lose weight and described eating less, taking more exercise and being successful at losing weight. They described how they wanted to show the practitioners running the service how they had changed their lifestyle in response to the advice received	Convergence Complementarity in that the qualitative research identifies why some people lost weight—they felt motivated to do so and felt that their progress was visible to someone they liked
Cholesterol	No change	No information	Silence
Smoking	No change	Practitioners described how patients who smoked often had no motivation to stop smoking. Patients in the qualitative sample who smoked described having no motivation to stop	Convergence Complementarity in that the qualitative research identifies the importance of motivation to change as a mechanism of impact
Diet	Improved	Some patients described eating less, especially if motivated to lose weight at the start of the RCT	Convergence Complementarity
Physical activity	Improved	Some patients described being motivated by the practitioners to take more exercise	Convergence Complementarity -the qualitative research shows the importance of the practitioner in facilitating change
Drug adherence	Improved	Some patients described being sent to their GP to discuss medication for high blood pressure	Convergence

(continued)

Table 11.1 Continued

Theme	RCT	Qualitative	Convergence, complementarity, contradiction, silence
Satisfaction with treatment and access to care	Improved	Some patients really liked the service and viewed it as filling a gap in provision. For others it was not perceived to be useful because they did not want to change their lifestyle	Convergence Complementarity - the qualitative research identified that some patients perceived a gap in service provision which the intervention filled, a contextual issue relevant to the potential effect of the intervention in other settings
Care coordination	Improved	Some patients wanted their GPs to take more interest in the intervention and their progress with it	Possible evidence of contradiction
Self management skills	No change	Some patients described how the intervention helped them to manage their health	Contradiction. Was the instrument used to measure this in the RCT too generic or did interviewees hold different definitions of self management from that measured in the RCT?
Quality of life	No change	Some patients described improvements in quality of life, in particular having more energy	Contradiction. Was the instrument used to measure this too generic? Or did this affect only a few people?
Further use of telehealth	No change	No mention of this	Silence or convergence because there was no discussion of this in the qualitative research and no sign of change in the RCT
Adverse events	One person in the intervention arm hospitalized for low blood pressure	An interviewee had returned to the GP with low blood pressure after losing weight	Convergence

Reproduced with courtesy of the author.

Source: data from Salisbury, C., et al. (2017) 'An evidence-based approach to the use of telehealth in long-term health conditions: development of an intervention and evaluation through pragmatic randomised controlled trials in patients with depression or raised cardiovascular risk'. *Programme Grants for Applied Research*, No. 5.1. Copyright © 2017.

- **The RCT has a small or modest effect and the qualitative findings show a feasible and acceptable intervention with some problems** around mechanism of impact, implementation or context. Here the journal article may focus on the mechanisms of action and how to address the problems to potentially improve the effect of the intervention in the future.
- **The RCT is null and the qualitative findings are about substantial problems** with the proposed mechanisms of action, implementation or context. Here the journal article may focus on how intervention developers can improve this type of intervention for future evaluation, or on the characteristics of an intervention that might prove to be more successful.

11.3.1.3 Partial agreement or disagreement

The qualitative research conclusions may not be fully aligned with the RCT result. The strength of the RCT is measurement of outcomes and the strength of the qualitative research is understanding processes. These different strengths must be held in mind at all times. There are two possible scenarios around partial agreement or disagreement of conclusions:

- **The RCT is null but in the qualitative research those delivering the intervention and those receiving are extremely positive about the intervention.** The research team needs to consider why this might be the case. They need to consider the quality of the RCT and the qualitative research, and the comparability of samples in each component. Moffatt et al. (2006) did this when they found a discrepancy between the qualitative research and the pilot RCT of an intervention offering welfare advice in general practice. Although the pilot RCT was not powered to show an effect, there was no evidence of change in any of the intermediate outcomes. Yet interviewees in the qualitative study discussed the importance of the extra funding they obtained from the welfare service to their quality of life. The research team considered a number of reasons for this discrepancy, including that the qualitative research might have sampled only from those with a positive experience. The conclusion they drew was that the discrepancy was most likely due to RCT participants receiving the welfare money after the primary outcome was measured in the pilot RCT because there was a longer than expected delay between referral to receive welfare and obtaining the money.
- **The RCT shows a large effect size but the qualitative research identifies significant problems with the intervention.** It can easily be the case that the intervention is so effective that even significant problems with its implementation may not overly diminish its impact. However, it is still worth considering why this discrepancy has occurred, again considering the

quality of the RCT and the qualitative research, and the comparability of samples in each component.

11.3.1.4 Explaining secondary outcomes: triangulation of findings

As well as explaining the overall RCT result, there is the option of using the qualitative research to explore why some secondary or intermediate outcomes were achieved or not. In the example in Box 10.1 in Chapter 10, although there was no change in the primary outcome in the RCT, there were reductions in self-reported consumption of high-energy drinks, snacks, and screen-viewing. The process evaluation shed light on these specific findings.

An adapted triangulation protocol can be used to help to explain changes in secondary outcomes in the RCT. An example of this is shown in Box 11.1, based on a set of published papers from a single study. An adapted triangulation protocol was not used in the study and therefore was not reported in any of these publications. This technique has been applied retrospectively for the purpose of displaying how it could be used. Application of the technique has two benefits. First, it produces an audit trail. Second, it can help researchers to approach integration methodically so that findings that agree are not favoured over those that disagree.

11.3.2 Exploring unusual findings from the RCT

An unusual finding may occur in an RCT, such as an increase in a secondary or primary outcome where a reduction was expected. It may be possible to explore the qualitative data that has already been collected to address this unusual finding, or to collect further qualitative data after the RCT outcome is known. Munro and Bloor (2010) discuss the challenge of being asked to explain an unusual finding in a pilot RCT. They did not have the time or money to undertake further qualitative research to explore an unusual finding in the RCT and this limited the confidence they had in their proposed explanation for the unusual finding. They caution against expectations that qualitative research or process evaluations can address any or all questions arising from an RCT.

11.3.3 Exploring discrepancies between the qualitative research and the RCT findings or data

As explained earlier in this Section 11.3.1, there is not always agreement between the qualitative and the RCT findings. This is also the case when considering the qualitative and quantitative data available on the same individuals. For example, Campbell et al. (2003) constructed a matrix comparing the change in the primary outcome in the RCT with perceived views of change in the primary outcome for individual patients interviewed in the concurrent qualitative study: that is, they

Box 11.2 Example of using triangulation protocol to compare qualitative and quantitative findings within a process evaluation of an RCT

Tonkin-Crine and colleagues (2016) undertook a process evaluation alongside a factorial cluster RCT of an intervention aiming to reduce antibiotic prescribing in general practice. The process evaluation consisted of surveys of 346 general practitioners (GPs) and 2886 patients in the RCT, and of qualitative interviews with 66 GPs and 62 patients in the intervention arms of the RCT. The findings from these four datasets were published in three peer-reviewed journal articles, reporting (1) the surveys, (2) the qualitative interviews with GPs, and (3) the qualitative interviews with patients. Then the team combined these findings using triangulation protocol to see if further insights could be gained. Three team members identified the key findings from each dataset in the form of statements summarizing each finding. These 74 findings were then compared to consider agreement, partial agreement, dissonance and silence between pairs of findings. The authors reported that triangulation protocol was easy to do and that it generated new findings and offered insights into the original findings. A new finding emerged from apparent dissonance between findings from the two qualitative datasets. GPs seemed to overestimate the need for a diagnostic test to convince patients that they did not need antibiotics because patients reported being happy with the GP opinion without the need for the diagnostic test.

Source: data from Tonkin-Crine, S., et al. and on behalf of the GRACE INTRO/CHAMP consortium. (2016). 'Discrepancies between qualitative and quantitative evaluation of randomised controlled trial results: achieving clarity through mixed methods triangulation'. *Implementation Science*, Issue 11, p. 66. Copyright © Tonkin-Crine et al. 2016.

used the matrix approach for integrating data that was described in Section 11.2.3. They found numerous discrepancies for individuals, raising the question of why this occurred. For example, some patients showed no change in their RCT primary outcome data but described large improvements in their health problem during their qualitative interview.

The main issue about discrepancy is not its identification but understanding why it has occurred. Fielding and Fielding (1986) call this 'apparent intermethod discrepancy' because there is likely to be an explanation for what appears to be a discrepancy. Exploring possible explanations can lead to further insights about the issue under study. Moffatt et al. (2006) display a thorough investigation of their apparent discrepancy between conclusions from their pilot RCT and qualitative research, with significant implications for their proposed full RCT. An example of exploring a discrepancy is displayed later in the Chapter in Box 11.2.

11.3.4 Combining the qualitative and quantitative findings from the process evaluation

Process evaluations can involve a number of data sets, including routine data on how much of the intervention each participant uses; data collected about processes as part of the RCT questionnaires, for example satisfaction with the intervention; surveys of practitioners delivering the intervention; non-participant observation of the intervention; and in-depth interviews with practitioners and patients. Triangulation protocol can be used to combine the findings from all these data sets (Integration B in Figure 11.3). Tonkin-Crine et al. (2016) describe in detail how they do this, including their approach to identifying key findings from each dataset and the teamwork to consider the relationship between findings from each dataset (see Box 11.2). Their study is described in more detail in Figure 9.1 in Chapter 9. They publish their convergence coding matrix in an appendix of the article; this acts as an audit trial and is useful for readers to consider when assessing the quality of the inferences drawn from this integration.

Any theory informing the intervention or the evaluation (see Chapter 6) may be used to structure the convergence coding matrix of themes, for example Normalization Process Theory. The functions of a process evaluation may also be used for this purpose, for example context, implementation, and mechanisms of impact (Moore et al. 2015) or fidelity, dose, reach (Linnen and Steckler, 2002).

11.3.5 Synthesizing findings from the whole evaluation

Triangulation protocol can be applied to a large number of datasets from the RCT and process evaluation (Integration C in Figure 11.3). Hutchings et al. (2016) have developed an alternative approach to triangulation protocol for this. They developed the approach because they did not find the published approaches useful for their complex evaluation. They call their approach MATRICS and applied it in the context of an evaluation with 10 methods including an RCT and qualitative research. Their approach requires the research team to identify three layers: first, all potential effects of the intervention, based on the aims and objectives of the study; second, all methods used in the evaluation; and third, all research findings. They show a worked example in their journal article.

11.3.6 Exploring variation in outcomes in the RCT

Oakley et al. (2006) show how a process evaluation can be used to explore the relationship between RCT outcomes and the extent and quality of the implementation of the intervention. In cluster RCTs some clusters can have larger effect sizes than others, leading to the question of why this has occurred. For example, Hoddinott et al. (2010) undertook a cluster RCT of breastfeeding in groups (see Box 4.3 in Chapter 4 for details of the study). They treated each cluster effect size from the RCT, and qualitative findings for a cluster, as a case within a multiple case study. They then considered how differences in staff attitudes and resources between the clusters could explain differences in the primary outcome of breastfeeding rates between those clusters. They did not display how they undertook this integration but it is likely that some form of matrix was used, displaying findings for each cluster.

It is helpful to plan to explore variation in outcomes before starting the study. This was not planned in an evaluation of evidence-based leaflets in maternity care and it was not possible to explore the variation in effect between the five clusters (O'Cathain et al., 2002) because the data for the concurrent ethnographic study (Stapleton et al. 2002) had not been collected and analysed in a way that facilitated such an analysis.

Similarly, in individual-level RCTs, some participants improve and others do not. Interviewees for the qualitative research can be selected by their level of response to the intervention after the RCT outcomes are known to explore why this variation occurred.

11.3.7 Qualitative research-generated subgroup analyses

Oakley et al. (2006) show how process evaluations can identify subgroup analyses for testing with the RCT data. In the published protocol for an RCT, researchers usually pre-specify a set of subgroup analyses. However, the qualitative research can generate further hypotheses prior to the RCT outcomes being known. This is a form of 'following a thread' described in Section 11.2.2. An example of this is shown in Box 11.3 which continues the example first introduced in Box 11.1.

11.3.8 Understanding moderators and mediators

Hypotheses generated from qualitative research can relate to moderators and mediators. A moderator is a variable that affects the relationship between two variables, such as a baseline covariate like age affecting the relationship between the intervention and the primary outcome. So in the example described

Box 11.3 An example of hypothesis generation, a form of 'following a thread'

The protocol for an evaluation of telehealth to reduce CVD risk factors (Thomas et al. 2014) specified that the outcome would be tested for differences by age, sex, baseline CVD risk and type of modifiable risk factor at baseline (high blood pressure, obesity, smoking status). It also stated that additional subgroups of interest might be identified by the process evaluation and that analysis of additional subgroups would be agreed upon with the Data Monitoring Committee and the Trial Steering Committee, with reporting of all analyses performed. In the published journal article of the RCT results, subgroup analyses identified no statistically significant results (Salisbury et al., 2016). This was due to lack of statistical power. There were indications of some differences: the odds ratio for people overweight at baseline was 1.7 compared with 1.1 for others. This indication of a difference by obesity was supported by the qualitative research which identified that people who joined the RCT with motivation to lose weight engaged with the intervention and reported taking action and losing weight. Similarly, the odds ratio for smokers was 1.1 compared with 1.4 for non-smokers; the qualitative research identified the lack of motivation of smokers to stop smoking or engage with the intervention. In the published report of the study, the qualitative research generated subgroup analyses which were then tested when the RCT outcomes were known (Salisbury et al., 2017). These were labelled as 'post hoc subgroup analyses as suggested by the embedded qualitative study' (p. 160). None were statistically significant. One analysis related to people with more severe problems being more likely to benefit from the intervention, that is, similar to the pre-specified subgroup analysis. There was some indication of this for weight loss as reported earlier in this Box. Another was that those with high levels of motivation to join the RCT would show better outcomes. The odds ratios were 1.3 and 1.4 for low and high internal motivation at baseline respectively, showing no indication of a difference. Another was that patients had to make considerable efforts to change their lifestyle whereas prescribed medication to reduce high blood pressure required less effort. The expectation was that the effect size would be higher for blood pressure than the lifestyle variables.

Source: data from Salisbury, C., et al. (2017) 'An evidence-based approach to the use of telehealth in long-term health conditions: development of an intervention and evaluation through pragmatic randomised controlled trials in patients with depression or raised cardiovascular risk'. *Programme Grants for Applied Research*, No 5.1. Copyright © 2017.

in Box 11.4 the potential moderator was educational status. A mediator does not affect the relationship between two variables but is on the causal pathway. For example, motivation to lose weight can affect weight loss in an RCT; a mediator is engagement with the intervention in that motivation affects engagement which affects impact on weight loss. Qualitative research can identify new mediators which are not documented within the theory or logic model of the intervention under evaluation, or challenge the importance of a mediator within the theory. Quantitative data collected as part of the RCT and process evaluation can then be used to explore mediators (Oakley et al., 2006; Emsley et al., 2010).

11.4 Challenges faced and potential solutions

Integration is not necessarily straightforward. Some of the challenges of doing this are explored and potential solutions offered where possible.

Box 11.4 An example of a hypothesis generated by the qualitative research, with exploration of a discrepancy in findings

The qualitative research undertaken alongside a pragmatic RCT identified a hypothesis that women with lower levels of education reported more benefit from a decision aid than those with higher levels of education (Protheroe et al., 2007). when this was tested in the RCT data, the opposite was found. The authors then explored this discrepancy in the discussion of their paper. They considered four possible explanations: that the quantitative analysis lacked statistical power, that the sample in the qualitative study was biased, that there were differences in interpretation of the outcome in women with different levels of education, and that there were different meanings of the outcome within the qualitative and RCT datasets. They concluded that the most likely explanation was different meanings of the outcome: the qualitative research identified that women with lower educational status reported being more empowered by the intervention and that the outcome measure used in the RCT had not measured empowerment.

Source: data from Protheroe, J., et al. (2007) 'The use of mixed methodology in evaluating complex interventions: identifying patient factors that moderate the effects of a decision aid'. *Family Practice*, Volume 24, Issue 6, pp. 594–600.

11.4.1 The credibility of the integration

When integration occurs, careful consideration will need to be given to the processes of integration. Researcher bias may be at play and this can be addressed in two ways.

- First, through transparency. It is important that a clear analysis plan is devised by the evaluation team, considering the approaches taken to integration and the timing of such integration. A detailed plan for integration may not be possible until the qualitative research has been analysed. Credibility may be gained from being clear that the qualitative data was analysed prior to the RCT results being known. This occurred in the examples in Boxes 10.1 and 11.1 and is put forward as a strength of a process evaluation of a school-based intervention to improve children's lifestyle (see Box 10.1). If hypotheses are generated for testing effectiveness in different subgroups it will be important to document that the timing of the generation of these hypotheses occurred prior to analysis of RCT data, and document the exact hypothesis. Formal submission of key qualitative research-generated sub group analyses to the Trial Steering Group will also facilitate transparency (see Chapter 15). Some of these subgroup analyses may have been pre-specified in the protocol and if so analysis will be undertaken anyway and the qualitative research can help to explain these quantitative findings. Even though these subgroup analyses are undertaken prior to analysis of the RCT, wider team members may view them as post hoc and insist that they are labelled in this way.
- Second, through reflective and critical engagement about any potential challenges around integration. For example, analyses can be accompanied by expressions of due caution. 'Following a thread' can occur until a researcher finds something statistically significant in the quantitative data set. The potential solution is to establish the analysis as exploratory and identify a clear hypothesis for further testing in another study. Engaging wider team members in discussion about plans, approaches and findings will help this reflection. It can help if a number of team members are involved in the integration. For example, three researchers who undertook the process evaluation worked as a team during integration, looking for consensus during the triangulation protocol (Tonkin-Crine et al., 2016).

11.4.2 Having the resources to integrate

Integration of any qualitative and quantitative data or findings occurs after analysis of both data sets. The 'third effort' of integration described in wider mixed methods research is relevant here (Morgan, 1998). Generating hypotheses for the RCT statisticians to test may be viewed as extra work and unwelcome at a busy time in the study for these statisticians. This resource issue can be addressed by planning integration at the start of the study with wider team members and building it into the workload and timetable of relevant team members.

11.4.3 Having the relevant quantitative data

A hypothesis can be generated from qualitative research but there may not be exact variables in the RCT data to test it. Instead, proxy variables may be tested. A problem with proxy variables is that if the finding is null then it is easy to explain this away as the proxy not accurately reflecting the issue identified in the qualitative research.

11.4.4 Having statistical power to test hypotheses

Where integration involves hypothesis generation and testing, there is unlikely to be the necessary statistical power within the quantitative data. This should not be viewed as a reason for not testing hypotheses. Sometimes there may be no sign of a relationship and sometimes there may be a sizeable difference in effect sizes between subgroups. This latter scenario has to be treated with caution but may lead to more confidence in pursuing that hypothesis in future studies.

11.4.5 Who does the integration

Integration may be difficult because some team members may not want to act on findings generated from the qualitative research. The findings may not be available at the time they are needed, the findings may not have credibility among some team members such as the lead researcher, the team running the RCT may be wedded to a particular path for their intervention and RCT and be unwilling to deviate from it, or the qualitative research may challenge established ways of thinking and practice. To facilitate integration, the whole evaluation team may need to adopt a reflexive approach associated with qualitative research (Hesse-Biber, 2012). This is discussed in more detail in Chapter 14.

11.4.6 Publication of integration

In the past, few studies combining qualitative research and RCTs reported explicit integration (Lewin et al. 2009). This may be due to structural issues associated with publication (see Chapter 12). Researchers may need to make explicit efforts to publish any integration they undertake. For the example in Box 11.1, the qualitative research was published in peer-reviewed journal articles after the two RCTs had been published. The title and abstract of the journal article reporting the qualitative findings made it clear that the purpose was to explain the findings of two RCTs (O'Cathain et al., 2016). The results of each RCT were summarized within the qualitative journal article (O'Cathain et al., 2016). However, the integration in terms of statistical analysis of qualitative research-generated subgroup analyses was reported in the final report only (Salisbury et al., 2017) and not in any subsequent journal article. This may have been due to the team running out of time to publish further journal articles, or a sense of not having an exciting story to tell because the statistical tests were null.

11.4.7 **Making causal inferences**

Qualitative research can help researchers to offer their best explanation for the results of an RCT. It cannot state that the causes of the RCT results. Attention to language is necessary to ensure that appropriate levels of uncertainty are communicated during any write up of the study.

11.5 Key points

- Integration includes taking actions from the qualitative research in the feasibility phase of a study to improve the full RCT procedures or intervention. The main challenge here is being transparent about how this integration occurred and who was involved with it.
- Integration can occur between the qualitative research and the RCT conclusions, findings, and data.
- Integration can occur within a process evaluation, as well as between the process evaluation and the RCT.
- Application of generic mixed methods integration techniques is useful.

11.6 **Questions to help you think about your study**

- What approaches to integration do you plan to take?
- Who needs to be involved in any integration and at what stage?
- Where will the insights from any integration be published?

Further reading

Farmer, T., Robinson, K., Elliott, S.J., Eyles, J. (2006). Developing and implementing a triangulation protocol for qualitative health research. *Qualitative Health Research*, **16**, pp. 377–394. doi: 10.1177/1049732305285708

Bazeley, P. (2009). 'Analysing mixed methods data' In: Andrew, S., Halcomb, E.J., (eds) *Mixed methods research for nursing and the health sciences*. Wiley-Blackwell, pp. 84–118.

O'Cathain, A., Murphy, E., Nicholl, J.P. (2010). Three techniques for integrating qualitative and quantitative methods in health services research. *BMJ*, **341**, pp. 1147–1150. doi: https://doi.org/10.1136/bmj.c4587.

Chapter 12

Publishing journal articles

Overview

Read this chapter to learn about

- Different combinations of publications from mixed methods evaluations
- Identifying the focus of a publication from the qualitative research
- Selecting a journal
- Guidance on key issues to include in publications
- Challenges and potential solutions

12.1 Introduction

The focus of this chapter is on reporting the qualitative research in peer-reviewed journal articles. Researchers may publish the qualitative data in a standalone journal article, or combine quantitative and qualitative process evaluation data in the same article, or combine the qualitative and RCT research in the same article. Writing these articles can be challenging, even when focusing solely on the qualitative research. Researchers need to consider the number of articles to be published from the whole study, the focus of an article, selecting a journal, and communicating implications for the RCT. Guidance is offered on the key issues to report in journal articles that focus solely on the qualitative research undertaken with an RCT.

12.2 Different combinations of publications

Approaches to publication can depend on the mixed methods design used for a study:

- In *sequential designs*, where the qualitative research is undertaken before the full RCT, publication of the qualitative research is likely to be in a separate journal article from the RCT and published prior to the RCT article. The conclusion of the qualitative research article can include explicit implications for the future RCT.

- In *concurrent designs*, where the qualitative research is undertaken alongside the full RCT, including as part of a process evaluation, researchers have a number of publication options available; these are described in Sections 12.2.1–12.2.4.

12.2.1 Mixed methods vs. monomethod publications

The qualitative research is sometimes published in the same article as the RCT (a mixed methods article). This tends to be undertaken in the context of a pilot RCT or a small single centre RCT. It is more usual to publish the qualitative research in a separate article from the RCT. This allows the researchers to offer the detail necessary to follow the CONSORT statement for reporting RCTs, and the detail necessary to describe the qualitative research. The downside of separate publications is that users of evidence of effectiveness may fail to link the separate articles unless researchers reference clearly between the articles. A mixed methods article may also be written based on the quantitative and qualitative research within a process evaluation.

12.2.2 A single vs. multiple publications

Multiple articles can be written from a single mixed methods evaluation (see Table 12.1). The RCT is usually published in a single journal article reporting the primary outcome and all the secondary outcomes. There can be other articles based on the RCT data, for example a mediation analysis showing the causal pathway of the intervention. Analysis within this mediation article may be shaped by findings from the qualitative research (see Chapter 11); that is, integration between qualitative and quantitative research can be described in such a publication. Similarly, the qualitative research can be published in a single article or multiple articles. A driver for publishing multiple articles from the qualitative research is that the research team want to report multiple stories or messages with different implications. Sometimes it is not possible to communicate all the key messages in a convincing way in a single publication. For example, there may be one message about mechanism of impact, showing how a key component of the intervention developed through the process of implementing the intervention, with implications for the transferability of the intervention outside the context of the RCT. There may be another message about the feasibility of delivering the intervention, with implications for explaining the RCT results (O'Cathain et al., 2013). This division of the qualitative research across a number of articles can be seen

Table 12.1 An example of the range of papers published from a single mixed methods evaluation of improving the lifestyles of school children (described in detail in Box 10.1 in Chapter 10).

Article	The focus of the publication	The data used	Timing	Journal	Integration	References to other articles from the study
1. Kipping et al. (2008)	Adapting the intervention to the UK	Pilot cluster RCT	2008	Archives of Disease in Childhood	Not applicable	Not applicable
2. Lawlor et al. (2011)	RCT protocol	None	2011	Trials	Qualitative research will help to understanding of how the intervention has any effect	1
3. Kipping et al. (2012)	Understanding acceptability and feasibility of adding a new component to the intervention	Qualitative research and quantitative process evaluation	2012	Journal of Public Health	Pilot RCT introduced as source of question about need for new component of intervention	1
4. Lawlor et al. (2013)	RCT statistical analysis plan	None	2013	Trials	Qualitative research not mentioned	2
5. Kipping et al. (2014)	RCT results	RCT data	2014	BMJ	Qualitative results from pilot referenced in discussion	1, 2, 3, 4
6. Jago et al. (2015)	Lessons for the future design of similar interventions	Process evaluation: parent and teacher interviews and child focus groups at end of intervention	2015	BMC Public Health	RCT result described in introduction	1, 2, 3, 4, 5, 7 (in review) Also the process evaluation plan published on the university website

(*continued*)

Table 12.1 Continued

Article	The focus of the publication	The data used	Timing	Journal	Integration	References to other articles from the study
7. Campbell et al. (2015)	Intervention fidelity	Qualitative and quantitative data from the process evaluation	2015	International Journal of Behavioral Nutrition and Physical Activity	Integration of findings In discussion shows convergence of RCT and process evaluation conclusions	2, 3, 4, 5, 6 Also states that findings from the process evaluation not included in this paper are reported elsewhere (forthcoming)
8. Lawlor et al. (2016a)	Mediator analysis	Quantitative data from RCT	2016	BMC Public Health	None. Could have considered relationship with qualitative findings	1, 2, 4, 5, 9 (in press)
9. Lawlor (2016b)	Full report of study	All data	2016	Public Health Research	All qualitative and quantitative findings reported together. Qualitative research shaped implications for future research.	All

Reproduced with courtesy of the author.

in the example in Table 12.1: one qualitative research article reports fidelity of the intervention with implications for explaining the result of the RCT, and the other reports implications for improving future interventions of that type. Another potential driver for publishing multiple articles is that there are multiple data sets. For example, interviews with practitioners delivering the intervention are published separately from interviews and focus groups with patients. This is likely to be a good publication strategy only if the key messages of the articles are different. Breaking the study up into too many pieces, or publishing different datasets separately because it seems an easy thing to do, may risk damaging communication of the key messages from the qualitative research.

12.2.3 Quantitative process data with the RCT or with the qualitative data

When quantitative and qualitative research are undertaken within a process evaluation, some of the quantitative data may be published in the RCT article, in particular the amount of the intervention used by RCT participants. The qualitative research from the process evaluation can be published separately. Alternatively both the qualitative and quantitative data from the process evaluation can be published in a mixed methods article. The decision will depend on the stories the researchers wish to tell.

12.2.4 Timing of publications—simultaneously vs. sequentially

The RCT and the qualitative research explaining the RCT results can be published in two separate articles side by side in the same journal, allowing readers of a single issue of a journal to read the articles together and undertake some implicit integration themselves. In the age of electronic searching for evidence, and electronic journals with continuous publication rather than weekly or monthly issues, this publication strategy may serve little purpose. It may also be challenging to deliver in practice because some journals publish RCTs but do not publish qualitative research.

It is more usual to publish the RCT and the qualitative research in different journals. In this scenario it is important to link the articles together clearly within each publication so that readers of the RCT article know there is a process evaluation or qualitative research explaining the results and can find the article easily. The sequencing of publication is important. If the qualitative research was undertaken to explain the findings of the RCT then it will be published after the RCT and refer to the RCT publication and result. In sequential publishing, sometimes one article needs to reference another that is not yet published. In the example in Table 12.1, the authors address this issue by referencing forthcoming articles in some of their publications.

Qualitative research can have implications for the RCT analysis or interpretation, or for future RCTs or similar interventions. It is important that these implications are central within the qualitative study publications, preferably in the abstract conclusions so that readers can see the importance and relevance of the findings to evidence of effectiveness. It is important that this integration (the implications of the qualitative research for the RCT) is explicit in publications, regardless of whether mixed methods or separate articles are published.

12.3 Identifying the focus of a publication

A publication from the qualitative research can rarely report all the issues identified in the analysis. The focus of an article or set of articles will be determined by consideration of the rationale for undertaking the qualitative research, the findings, and the unique contribution to knowledge. In one study, a key issue for explaining the RCT result may be that practitioners could not implement the intervention with fidelity. In another study, a key issue may be the potential importance of an intervention component to obtaining an effect. Articles that attempt to include a large number of themes risk offering a shallow analysis. Articles that focus on a single or small number of issues may be able to help those using evidence to really understand a key issue about how or why an intervention does or does not work.

12.4 Selecting a journal

A few years ago around a hundred journal articles a year were published from the qualitative research undertaken with RCTs (O'Cathain et al., 2013). Researchers published this work in a wide variety of journals, a list of which was published (O'Cathain et al., 2014b). The selection of a journal for publishing the qualitative research can depend on

- whether a journal publishes qualitative research (some do not),
- the audience a researcher wishes to reach (e.g., an article about an intervention to reduce depression can be placed in a mental health journal),
- the academic discipline of the researcher (some researchers can enhance their careers or reputation within their research community by publishing in sociology or psychology journals, although some of these journal may not publish the more applied qualitative research that can be undertaken with RCTs (O'Cathain et al., 2014a), or
- the reputation of a journal within a field or academic discipline.

12.5 Guidance on key issues to include in a publication

When publishing an article based only on the qualitative research from a mixed methods evaluation, researchers can follow COREQ reporting guidelines for qualitative research (Tong et al., 2007). However, there are further considerations when qualitative research has been undertaken with RCTs. An analysis of journal articles based on the qualitative research undertaken with RCTs resulted in production of guidance for reporting such articles: QUAlitative Research with Trials: Excellent Reporting (O'Cathain et al., 2014b). This guidance has been further developed into QUARTER2 for this book (see Table 12.2). It can be used in addition to, and not instead of, standard reporting guidance or guidelines for qualitative research (Tong et al., 2007).

When publishing a mixed methods article, guidance called Good Reporting of A Mixed Methods Study (GRAMMS) can be used (O'Cathain et al., 2008). Researchers may also wish to use QUARTER2 for the qualitative component of a mixed methods article.

12.6 Challenges faced and potential solutions

Even though there are around a hundred journal articles reporting the qualitative research undertaken with RCTs published annually in international journals (O'Cathain et al., 2013) a qualitative interview study of researchers in the UK who had led the RCT or qualitative research in a mixed methods evaluation, identified publication as an issue with considerable challenges (O'Cathain et al., 2014a). Interviewees identified structural issues at play which affect priorities for publication; these are discussed.

12.6.1 The differing status of qualitative and RCT publications

RCTs may be published in highly regarded journals, leading to these articles being viewed as prestigious by a researcher's organization and research community. However, the 'big' medical journals often do not accept qualitative research. These articles may therefore be published in what are perceived to be less prestigious journals. A recent social media campaign challenged the position adopted by a leading medical journal of not publishing qualitative research (Greenhalgh et al., 2016). The journal editors took this stance because they argued that qualitative research is not highly cited and does not have the impact of quantitative research (Loder et al., 2016). The example described in Box 1.1 in Chapter 1 offers evidence that contradicts this position by showing the impact of combining qualitative research and RCTs: the qualitative research identified problems with an existing service and shaped the changes made to a new

Table 12.2 Guidance for reporting qualitative research in journal articles: QUAlitative Research with Trials: Excellent Reporting version 2 (QUARTER2)

Focus of the article	Consider selecting a focus rather than trying to report all the findings. A single message powerfully told can have more meaning than several briefly described
Rationale for the research question	Explain the rationale of the focus of the article. Why is the focus important, how did it emerge and when did it emerge in relation to the RCT. This offers context to the findings. State the rationale in the abstract e.g. to explain the RCT result
Clarity of aim of the analysis presented in the article	Be clear about the aim of the analysis of the article both in the abstract and main body of the article. Sometimes research starts with a broad aim of 'exploring the views of patients' but the focused analysis for the article is the 'feasibility of the intervention' (see Chapter 8). Making this clear helps the reader understand the findings
Evaluation design	Place the research within the overall study design using mixed methods designs or an evaluative framework such as the MRC framework for the development and evaluation of complex interventions (see Chapter 2)
RCT	Describe the RCT, considering the information that is relevant to the qualitative research. If the rationale is to explain the RCT result then summarize the RCT result in the abstract and body of the article. Use the RCT acronym if it exists. This allows readers to connect journal articles from the same study and consider the implications for a specific RCT. The rationale also offers key context for the qualitative research and may affect its interpretation
Sampling	Describe whether the qualitative research was undertaken with participants experiencing the intervention or the control or both of these groups (see Chapter 9)
Data collection	Describe when the qualitative data collection was undertaken e.g. half way through the intervention, at the end of the intervention, after the primary outcome was measured.
Analysis	Describe when the qualitative analysis was undertaken and whether this was before the RCT results were known (see Chapter 10)
Balance	Give the qualitative research space in mixed methods articles
Conclusions and implications	Report implications for the specific RCT and future RCTs in both the abstract and the discussion. Make the implications for different stakeholders clear: trialists, intervention developers, service providers, and patients
References	Reference previous and forthcoming articles from the mixed methods evaluation to allow readers to find this evidence and understand how the current article fits within the evidence generated by the whole study

Reproduced with courtesy of the author.

service that saved many lives in different countries. Qualitative research can have an impact in combination with RCTs and it is important that this is recognized by research communities (see Chapter 16 for further discussion of the impact of qualitative research) and that journal editorial policies of excluding qualitative research continue to be challenged.

12.6.2 It is not published

The qualitative research undertaken with RCTs may not be published in peer-reviewed journal articles (Lewin et al., 2009). This may be because these articles are not a priority for the team—the RCT article is often described as the 'main paper'—or because the externally funded researcher leaves the study early to move on to another project, or all members of the team may move to the next set of studies and do not have time to publish what are perceived as the less important articles (O'Cathain et al., 2014b). Researchers may also face the challenge of writing an article that is different from the types of articles they usually see in journals, particularly if they have undertaken qualitative research in preparation for an RCT. Qualitative research undertaken in the development phase may be more difficult to write because of the iterative nature of the process of intervention development. A possible solution when faced with this challenge is to search for a few similar articles prior to writing and make use of the QUARTER2 guidance described in Section 12.5. It is usually important to publish the qualitative research because it is likely to have implications for future RCTs of similar interventions.

12.6.3 Getting the timing right

Sequential publication from a mixed methods evaluation was described in Section 12.2. The challenges of getting the sequence right, and not delaying one publication too long in order for another to be published first, may tempt researchers to publish articles from the qualitative research that make no reference to the RCT is any substantial way. A potential solution to this challenging issue is for the research team to develop a publication strategy early in the study and review this strategy throughout the project so the qualitative research can be published as quickly as possible with explicit messages either for the RCT it was undertaken with or for future RCTs.

12.6.4 A lack of expertise

Journal articles are not easy to write. Articles based on qualitative research undertaken with RCTs face particular challenges because they are related to another publication. The articles based on the qualitative research may be left to junior qualitative researchers to write, some of whom can produce high-quality publications and some of whom may struggle to write convincing articles. Contrast this with the RCT article which is usually first authored by the lead investigator, who is usually a senior researcher. Extensive involvement of senior qualitative expertise may help to ensure high-quality publications.

12.6.5 Writing a mixed methods article

If researchers choose to combine the RCT and qualitative research in a single journal article, this can produce challenges around the order of presentation of methods and findings, and the voice used within the article (O'Cathain, 2009). There is guidance available for reporting general mixed methods research (O'Cathain et al., 2008) that may help researchers.

12.7 Key points

- A range of publications can be produced from a single mixed methods evaluation, including qualitative articles and mixed methods articles.
- Qualitative research is undertaken in this context to be of value to generating evidence of effectiveness. Implications for the specific RCT and future RCTs can be made explicit in article abstracts.
- The guidance 'QUAlitative Research with Trials: Excellent Reporting' version 2 (QUARTER2) can be used to improve reporting of articles.
- Some high profile journals do not publish qualitative research. This can have implications for the resources given to publishing the qualitative research. It is important to publish the qualitative research if it has implications for the evidence of effectiveness of an intervention.

12.8 Questions to help you think about your study

- What are the key messages from the qualitative research? Do these have different implications for different audiences? What implications does this have for the numbers of journal articles to be published?
- Are members of your wider team willing to develop a publications strategy for the RCT and qualitative research, including timing of different publications?

Further reading

Tong, A., Sainsbury, P., Craig, J. (2007). Consolidated criteria for reporting qualitative research (COREQ): a 32-item checklist for interviews and focus groups. *International Journal for Quality in Healthcare*, **19**(6), pp. 349–357. doi: https://doi.org/10.1093/intqhc/mzm042.

Chapter 13

Assessing the quality of qualitative research undertaken with RCTs

Overview

Read this chapter to learn about

- Undertaking high quality qualitative research with RCTs
- How to assess quality

13.1 Introduction

In this chapter the focus is on how researchers can attend to quality when undertaking qualitative research with RCTs, including the steps involved in achieving methodological rigour. The assessment of the quality of published qualitative research is considered, and the range of guidance available presented.

13.2 Who assesses quality and when

The quality of mixed methods research in health is assessed by many stakeholders at different time points (O'Cathain et al., 2010; Curry and Nunez, 2015). These stakeholders focus on different aspects of quality:

- Funding bodies and reviewers assess grant proposals to consider whether to fund the research. They focus on whether the research question is important (utility), the research can be completed on time (feasibility), the methods are appropriate (methodological rigour), the research is ethical (ethics), and the research is value for money (economics). Researchers planning studies pay attention to these issues in order to produce high quality grant proposals.
- Once funded, researchers address the methodological rigour of their research and may self-assess this as they progress through their study.

- Reviewers, health practitioners and patients assess final reports and published journal articles for methodological rigour and relevance.
- Systematic reviewers critically appraise journal articles for inclusion or interpretation in evidence syntheses.

Methodological rigour is relevant to all stakeholders so this is considered further in this chapter.

13.3 Methodological rigour

Four steps are proposed for achieving methodological rigour of the qualitative research undertaken with RCTs.

13.3.1 Step 1: Use strategies for undertaking good quality qualitative research

Different research communities have their own meanings of quality of qualitative research and how to achieve and assess it. These meanings are shaped by the underlying research paradigm within that community, the philosophical stance adopted within the research study, and the values and beliefs of the academic disciplines of the researchers undertaking the qualitative research (such as nursing or psychology). External reviewers of reports and journals articles will apply their own beliefs and values, either implicitly or explicitly, when judging the quality of the qualitative research. This means that the meaning of quality is contested, with no consensus about strategies for achieving quality. A range of strategies have been identified in the context of qualitative research in health care (Pope and Mays, 2006), including triangulation, member checking, transparency of data collection and analysis, reflexivity, and attention to negative cases. Researchers undertaking qualitative research with RCTs can adopt these strategies. Examples of some of these strategies employed by researchers proposing or reporting qualitative research with RCTs in journal articles are shown in Box 13.1).

13.3.2 Step 2: Use strategies specific to a paradigm or approach taken

For example, if a participatory approach is taken to the mixed methods evaluation, then attend to any strategies for undertaking good quality participatory research.

13.3.3 Step 3: Consider relevant guidance on undertaking qualitative research with RCTs

There is guidance available on how to undertake process evaluations, both generally and more specifically, for cluster RCTs (Table 13.1). Qualitative research

Box 13.1 Examples of how researchers have reported attending to the quality of the qualitative research undertaken with RCTs in journal articles

PROTOCOL: Jack and colleagues (2015) published a protocol for the process evaluation of their evaluation of family nurse partnership in Canada (described in Box 8.2 in Chapter 8). They report a section called 'Rigour' in their protocol. They outline in a Table a number of strategies they will use to achieve credibility, dependability, and confirmability in their process evaluation. These include reflexivity, investigator triangulation, and dense description of methods to produce an audit trail.

PROTOCOL: Wiart and colleagues (2016) published a protocol for an RCT and qualitative research of gait training for young people with cerebral palsy in Canada (described in Boxes 2.1 and 8.1). For the qualitative component they report a section called 'enhancing credibility'. They describe four approaches to this, including methodological triangulation, maximum variation in all samples, an audit trail and peer review whereby preliminary analysis is presented to wider members of the team for critical feedback.

STUDY: Hoddinott and colleagues (2010) published the findings of qualitative research undertaken alongside an RCT of a breastfeeding intervention in the UK (described in Box 4.3 in Chapter 4). They report a separate section labelled 'validation and trustworthiness' where they describe paying attention to negative cases, using member checking on summaries of interviews, and using peer review of data collection and analysis by an external researcher.

STUDY: Bosch and colleagues (2016) published an article reporting a qualitative study to inform an RCT of managing patients with brain injuries in emergency departments in Australia (see Box 6.1 in Chapter 6). They did not have a separate section on quality but noted in the wider text that they produced an audit trail in their analysis by keeping a record of coding decisions.

is usually a key component of process evaluations. There is also guidance available for the more specific endeavour of undertaking qualitative research with RCTs, in particular within feasibility studies, and for writing proposals and publications. The available guidance is summarized in Table 13.1, with references cited to help readers locate the guidance easily. Some issues related to methodological rigour that are specific to qualitative research with RCTs have already been discussed throughout this book. In particular they are considered in Table 12.2 in Chapter 12, where guidance on reporting the qualitative

Table 13.1 List of available guidance relevant to qualitative research and RCTs

Focus of the guidance	Source
Process evaluations (see Chapter 2)	Moore, G., Audrey, S., Barker, M., Bond, L., Bonell, C., Cooper, C., Hardeman, W., Moore, L., O'Cathain, A., Tannaze, T., Wight, D., Baird, J. (2015). Process evaluation of complex interventions. Medical Research Council guidance. BMJ, 350, h1258. doi: 10.1136/bmj.h1258
Process evaluations for cluster RCTs (see Chapter 4)	Grant, A., Treweek, S., Dreischulte, T., Foy, R., Guthrie, B. (2013). Process evaluations for cluster-randomized trials of complex interventions: a proposed framework for design and reporting. Trials, 14, 15. doi: 10.1186/1745-6215-14-15
Using qualitative research in feasibility studies for RCTs (see Chapter 4)	O'Cathain, A., Hoddinott, P., Lewin, S., Thomas, K.J., Young, B., Adamson, J., Jansen, Y.J.F.M., Mills, N., Moore, G., Donovan, J.L. (2015). Maximizing the impact of qualitative research in feasibility studies for randomized controlled trials: guidance for researchers. Feasibility and Pilot Studies, 1, 32. doi: 10.1186/s40814-015-0026-y
Writing a research proposal for qualitative research with RCTs (see Chapter 7)	Drabble, S.J., O'Cathain, A., Thomas, K.J., Rudolph, A., Hewison, J. (2014). Describing qualitative research undertaken with randomized controlled trials in grant proposals: a documentary analysis. BMC Medical Research Methodology, pp. 14-24. doi: 10.1186/ 1471-2288-14-24
Reporting a publication from qualitative research and RCTs (QuaRTER 2) (see Chapter 12)	O'Cathain, A., Thomas, K.J., Drabble, S.J., Rudolph, A., Goode, J., Hewison, J. (2014b). Maximizing the value of combining qualitative research and randomized controlled trials in health research: the QUAlitative Research in Trials (QUART) study – a mixed methods study. Health Technology Assessment, 18(38), pp. 1–197. doi: 10.3310/hta18380

Reproduced with courtesy of the author.

research is described. For example, it is good practice to report the timing of analysing the qualitative research in relation to knowing the RCT result. The utility of guidance for reporting qualitative research with RCTs goes beyond simply facilitating transparent publications that allow readers to assess quality. Researchers can read reporting guidance before planning their study so they can attend to issues they want to report, thus improving the quality of their research as well as the reporting of it.

13.3.4 Step 4: Consider approaches to quality assessment of mixed methods research

If the qualitative research is published in the same article as quantitative research, then aspects of the reporting quality for mixed methods articles (O'Cathain et al., 2008) or quality criteria for mixed methods research can be applied (O'Cathain et al., 2010; Curry and Nunez-Smith, 2015; Fabregues and Molina-Azorin, 2016). Fabregues and Molina-Azorin (2016) detail a list of 19 commonly articulated items for assessing mixed methods research, ordered within four study phases.

13.4 Critically appraising a journal article

Stakeholders often want to judge the quality of the research reported in a journal article before they decide to take action on the findings, or include it in a systematic review (see Section 13.5). The Critical Appraisal Skills Programme (CASP) at http://www.casp-uk.net/casp-tools-checklists has produced a critical appraisal tool for use when reading qualitative research. The tool is short (ten items) and written in plain language to facilitate its use by a variety of stakeholders. The CASP tool can be applied to journal articles reporting qualitative research used with RCTs but is best applied after reading the guidance on reporting qualitative research undertaken with RCTs so that issues specific to this endeavour are considered within the more overarching items of CASP (see Table 13.1). For example, CASP includes an item about having a clear statement of aims. This is highly relevant given the problems with articulating aims clearly when reporting qualitative research with RCTs (see Chapter 12). Additionally, CASP ends with an item about the value of the research, including whether the researchers have considered the contribution it makes to current knowledge and transferability of the findings. Again, this is highly relevant because researchers sometimes fail to articulate the contribution the qualitative research has made to the specific RCT, future RCTs and the endeavour of assessing effectiveness (O'Cathain et al., 2014b).

13.5 Inclusion in systematic reviews

It is important to publish the qualitative research undertaken with RCTs so that others can learn from it. Once published, other researchers may consider its inclusion in systematic reviews and assess its quality as part of this endeavour. Qualitative research undertaken alongside RCTs can be brought together to help to explain the heterogeneity of RCT results of a specific type of intervention or for a specific patient group (Noyes et al., 2011). Or it can be brought together with all the research that contributes to understanding a specific complex intervention (Petticrew et al., 2013). The quality of the qualitative research will usually be formally assessed and this assessment is most likely to be used during interpretation of findings rather than to exclude poor quality studies. Ways of assessing the confidence that can be placed in any synthesis of qualitative research has also been considered (Lewin et al., 2015).

13.6 Key points

- A four-step process is proposed for attending to quality of the qualitative research undertaken with RCTs: (1) use well-known strategies for achieving quality for qualitative research, (2) use strategies associated with the research paradigm adopted, (3) consider published guidance on undertaking qualitative research with RCTs, and (4) consider approaches to achieving quality described in the wider mixed methods literature.
- Use the Critical Appraisal Skills Programme (CASP) checklist for appraising the quality of qualitative research after reading guidance on how to undertake qualitative research in this context.

13.7 Questions to help you think about your study

- When planning your study, which strategies will you adopt to attend to the quality of the qualitative research? Do you want to articulate this in your proposal or published protocol?
- When writing up your qualitative research, have you been transparent about its relationship with the RCT?

Further reading

Fàbregues, S., Molina-Azorín, J.F. (2016). Addressing quality in mixed methods research: A review and recommendations for a future agenda. *Quality & Quantity*, pp. 1–17. doi: 10.1007/s11135-016-0449-4.

Part 3

Engaging relevant stakeholders

Chapter 14

Team working

Overview

Read this chapter to learn about

- Different team configurations
- The importance of communicating and reflecting on team members' world views
- Team involvement in planning the study
- When and how to share the qualitative findings
- Type of team working that maximizes the value of the qualitative research

14.1 Introduction

The focus of this chapter is on team work. How a team works together can affect the value of the qualitative research for the RCT and the generation of evidence of effectiveness of the intervention. How a team works best together may depend on the phase of the study—whether it is a feasibility study or the full evaluation—and the timing of completion of the qualitative research in relation to the full RCT.

14.2 Team configurations

Different configurations of teams are possible in studies combining qualitative research and RCTs. This can have implications for the qualitative research:

- Sometimes a research team works as **a series of sub-teams**, with the full team meeting a few times a year to report on progress of data collection and analysis from the different sub-teams. Each sub-team may have separate responsibility for the qualitative research, the economic modelling and the RCT. In this team configuration, the lead investigator is often the lead for the RCT. The focus of this chapter is on the wider team rather than the qualitative sub-team. The wider team may include triallists or clinical trials unit staff, qualitative researchers, statisticians, the intervention developer, clinicians, public and patient involvement representatives, and economists.

- An alternative configuration is a **whole-team approach**, where the wider team meets regularly with a commitment to sharing ongoing findings as well as progress with data collection. In some scenarios the lead investigator of the whole study may lead both the RCT and the qualitative research.

In the first configuration it may be very difficult for wider team members to engage with the qualitative research and understand the implications of any findings for their parts of the study unless efforts are made to communicate findings when appropriate. In the second configuration it may be difficult to manage the timing of communicating qualitative findings so that the RCT experiment is not compromised. These issues are discussed in more detail later in the chapter.

14.3 Understanding the different world views of each team member

Different team members can hold different world views in terms of having different beliefs and values about how to undertake research. This is often referred to as having different research paradigms or epistemological positions. Indeed an interesting aspect of combining qualitative research and RCTs within mixed methods studies is the extremes of epistemological positions that each are associated with (see Chapter 5). Even where combining methodologies is normal within research communities, there may be the potential for conflict, misunderstanding, benign dismissal of different methodologies, or lost opportunities for integration unless team dynamics are explicitly addressed.

In any mixed methods study, team members attempting to work in an interdisciplinary way each bring with them a range of identities related to gender, age, ethnicity, academic discipline, methods expertise, and status in the workplace (Curry et al., 2012). To facilitate productive team working, teams may need to spend time actively communicating individuals' beliefs and values, while also understanding the range of identities people bring to the team. Curry et al. (2012) recommend paying attention to letting different experts in the team be different, building trust as a group, ensuring time and processes for information sharing, and offering inclusive leadership.

As discussed in Chapter 15, some team members can be invested in the intervention or the RCT to such an extent that they find it difficult to listen to any emerging findings that challenge their beliefs, and therefore find it difficult to take actions from the qualitative research that involve changing the intervention or the RCT design or conduct. This could include the qualitative researcher who may have been involved in developing the intervention and exploring its feasibility and acceptability in earlier phases of the evaluation. Team reflexivity and team communication are required here.

Teams can develop an understanding over the history of a single study or over a series of studies as they accumulate knowledge about team members and the strengths of different methods and methodologies.

14.4 **Planning the study together**

A key finding of qualitative interview studies undertaken with mixed methods researchers (O'Cathain et al., 2008) and qualitative and RCT researchers (O'Cathain et al., 2014a) was the importance of qualitative researchers planning the evaluation together with other team members at the proposal writing stage. Integrated working at this planning stage can result in qualitative research being used in the right places for the right purpose and with enough resource to ensure that high-quality qualitative research is undertaken.

14.5 **Sharing findings between team members during the research**

Team working is of such importance when combining qualitative research and RCTs that Moore et al. (2015) in their process evaluation guidance present a box outlining the arguments for separating or integrating the teams delivering the process and outcome evaluations. Decision-making around separation versus integration of teams may depend on the study phase, the purpose of the qualitative research, and the timing of completion of different tasks within a full evaluation.

14.5.1 **Feasibility phase**

In feasibility studies for RCTs, a dynamic or iterative approach to qualitative research is recommended whereby qualitative research is undertaken early in the feasibility study and the findings fed back to the wider team so that actions can be undertaken to improve the intervention or the RCT conduct if deemed necessary (O'Cathain et al., 2015). Then further qualitative research can be undertaken to check if problems identified have been addressed and identify further problems. Quantitative process data may also be used to check whether problems have been fixed, for example recruitment rates have increased or more patients are using the intervention. Here, close team working is essential, with intervention developers and triallists open to hearing the findings of the qualitative research and thinking about the actions to take during the feasibility study. Given that the primary health outcome is not the focus of any pilot RCT within a feasibility study, concerns about damaging the RCT experiment are unlikely to be warranted. An important ethical issue to consider during this dynamic ongoing feedback of qualitative findings is the protection of the anonymity of interviewees (Cooper et al., 2014). Qualitative researchers may also have to work at taking a different approach to analysis, learning to be comfortable with rapid transcription and preliminary analysis while taking care not to be over confident about early findings.

An alternative approach is for the RCT and qualitative sub-teams to work separately and wait until the end of the feasibility study to feed back any qualitative findings to the whole team. A disadvantage of this approach is that the team have to make decisions to change the intervention or RCT conduct without having any information about whether these actions result in improvements in processes. It is also the case that teams sometimes disperse at the end of studies and this valuable stage of feedback and action planning may be lost. Alternatively the team may be in a position to proceed to the full RCT as soon as they have completed the feasibility study. If this is the case then an appropriate length of time is needed between the feasibility study and the full RCT to allow time for the qualitative analysis and any changes to be made to the intervention.

Regardless of whether feedback of qualitative findings is ongoing throughout the feasibility study or left to the end, wider team members will have to consider what actions to take and when because this qualitative research may identify a large number of issues that could be addressed. An approach to this, developed by Bugge et al. (2013), is discussed in Chapter 16.

14.5.2 Evaluation phase

In the evaluation phase, when and where to communicate findings from the qualitative research requires more thought because of concerns that feeding back findings from the qualitative research while the full RCT is in progress could have detrimental effects on the RCT (Cooper et al., 2014). Here, researchers need to be clear about the purpose of the qualitative research and subsequently the appropriate timing of communicating the findings to the wider team.

- **A purpose to improve intervention implementation.** Researchers can undertake qualitative research during the full RCT with an aim of exploring the intervention implementation. The content of the intervention will be fixed during this phase but there may be aspects of how the intervention is delivered that the team is happy to change as the RCT progresses (Hawe et al., 2004). For example, it may be acceptable to change any large problems with intervention delivery during an internal pilot RCT. However, such changes need to undertaken with care and documented so the team can be transparent when reporting the RCT. Qualitative researchers will need to plan what to feed back to the wider team and who should be part of this team. Feedback of problems with the intervention to a team that includes the recruiters for the RCT may lead to demoralization of those recruiters and subsequent reduction in efforts to recruit (Cooper et al., 2014). Communicating problems with the intervention to a team that includes staff delivering the intervention may lead to undocumented changes to the intervention or its delivery, undermining the premise that the RCT is evaluating a fixed intervention throughout the RCT. Here, the wider team needs to discuss the pros and cons of feeding back during recruitment, or during intervention delivery, and consider who should be present during feedback sessions.

- **A purpose to improve RCT conduct.** When full RCTs struggle with recruitment the lead investigator may consider using the QUINTET intervention of qualitative research to identify reasons for recruitment difficulties and associated solutions (Donovan et al., 2016). Here, the wider team needs to listen to feedback from the qualitative research and take actions to make the RCT viable in terms of recruitment to target.
- **A purpose to explain RCT results.** At the end of the qualitative research or process evaluation, it is good practice to analyse the data before the RCT results are known (Moore et al., 2015; Oakley et al., 2006). As Moore et al. (2015) point out, this may not always be possible if the process evaluation is complex and requires a long time to analyse. If researchers complete the qualitative research before the RCT has completed recruitment or intervention delivery, qualitative researchers may wish to feed back findings to the wider team or publish an early journal article. If the qualitative findings are negative about the intervention then this may cause demoralization of recruiters or change the behaviour of those delivering the intervention (Cooper et al., 2014) so the timing of feedback needs careful consideration. Feedback when the intervention delivery is complete, or at the end of the RCT when the RCT outcome is known, is far less problematic. At this point the wider team needs to be open to the findings so they can consider the interpretation of the RCT results. A challenge here is that qualitative researchers may not still be employed on the team at this stage (Cooper et al., 2014). It may also be helpful for the quality of the qualitative research to engage the wider team in helping to interpret the qualitative research. For example, Audry et al. (2006) describe a sub-group of the research team that took primary responsibility for the process evaluation but all members of the

team, which included statisticians, social scientists and health promotion specialists, were encouraged to comment before the process evaluation was finalized. This level of involvement of the wider team is likely to facilitate the use of the qualitative research to interpret the RCT results.

Researchers have also expressed concern when there is overlap between members of the RCT and the process evaluation teams (Liu et al., 2016). They see this as a strength in that the process evaluation team fully understand the RCT but also as a weakness in terms of introducing bias into the process evaluation because of a desire to view the intervention and RCT in a positive light.

14.6 **Working to obtain maximum value from the qualitative research**

A qualitative interview study of researchers undertaking mixed methods studies in the UK identified team working as a key issue facilitating or hindering integration of the qualitative and quantitative components of a study (O'Cathain et al., 2008). Teams were characterized as dysfunctional, multidisciplinary, or interdisciplinary, with the last type open to respectful communication focused on a desire to learn from other methods within the study and thus more likely to undertake integration. A similar qualitative interview study of researchers working on mixed methods evaluations involving qualitative research and RCTs in the UK identified a related set of three models of relationship of the qualitative research to the RCT (O'Cathain et al., 2014a):

- The first model was '*the peripheral*', where the RCT simply offered qualitative researchers an opportunity to undertake their research and there was no intention that it would be of value to the RCT or the endeavour of generating evidence of effectiveness. Here, qualitative researchers used the RCT context to recruit interviewees and explore a health problem such as diabetes, sometimes for a formal qualification such as a PhD. This chapter is not relevant to this context.
- The second model was '*the add-on*', where the qualitative researcher understood the potential value of the qualitative research to the RCT but their work was viewed as a separate and complementary endeavour by the wider team. The wider team viewed the RCT as the study, and did not see the qualitative research as something that would change how they undertook or interpreted the RCT. Interviewees described how this could limit the value of the qualitative research to the RCT. In the worse cases the qualitative research or process evaluation was seen as a token gesture to appease funders who wanted this study component included alongside the RCT. This model has also been identified in the USA (Song et al., 2010)

- The third model was '*the integral*', which operated in two ways. Within this model the lead investigator of the whole study viewed the qualitative research as an essential part of the evaluation due to the complexity of the intervention or context in which the evaluation occurred, and due to uncertainties about the intervention or RCT conduct that qualitative research could address. These lead investigators described being driven by the need to undertake research which was applicable to the complex world in which health and health care operates and how they could not conceive of undertaking an RCT of the types of issues they were interested in without also using qualitative research. Some of these teams appeared to be 'integral in theory' because the qualitative research was under-resourced. In contrast, 'integral in practice' teams planned the qualitative research from the beginning of the study, had senior qualitative expertise on the team from beginning to end, and had dedicated staff and time to deliver the research. That is, these teams invested resources in the qualitative research because they valued it. Interviewees from this latter type of team described the value of the qualitative research to the RCT in practice, for example they changed their outcome measure for the full RCT or understood why an intervention did or did not work.

14.7 Key points

- Team working can be improved if team members reflect together on the different world views held by team members.
- Consideration is needed of when best to feed back the findings of the qualitative research to the wider team. Ongoing feedback can be useful in feasibility studies for RCTs but care is needed when practising this in the context of the full RCT.
- Qualitative research studies of tram working suggests that the value of qualitative research when used with RCTs is maximized if lead investigators believe that the qualitative research is integral to the evaluation, and give it the resources it needs to deliver good quality research.

14.8 Questions to help you think about your study

- What are the pros and cons of feeding back findings of the qualitative research to the wider team at different times during your study?
- When you talk about the qualitative research in the wider team are all members actively engaged? That is, are they considering how your work might

help them to improve the intervention, the RCT conduct, the RCT analysis or the RCT interpretation?

- Does your team need some meetings to get to know each other's beliefs about research, and who is invested in the intervention or RCT and how to manage this?

Further reading

O'Cathain, A., Goode, J., Drabble, S.J., Thomas, K.J., Rudolph, A., Hewison, J. (2014a). Getting added value from using qualitative research with randomised controlled trials: a qualitative interview study. *Trials*, **15**, 215. doi: 10.1186/1745-6215-15-215.

Chapter 15

Engaging with key stakeholders

Overview

Read this chapter to think about how best to engage with different groups of people who may be external to the evaluation team. Learn about engagement with

- People who may have a vested interest in the intervention under evaluation (e.g., intervention developers and policy makers)
- Groups that offer oversight of research (e.g., trial steering committees)
- Ethics committees
- Patient and public involvement

15.1 **Introduction**

A range of stakeholders can interact with the qualitative research undertaken with RCTs. Some may be part of the evaluation team (patient and public involvement definitely, intervention developers possibly), but most are external to the team (e.g., members of trial steering committees). It is important to think about these stakeholders and plan their interaction with the qualitative research to ensure the best qualitative research is undertaken, and that findings from the qualitative research are acted upon.

15.2 **Working with intervention developers and policy makers**

The evaluation team may work closely with the intervention developers or policy makers keen to implement an intervention. Both of these stakeholders may lack equipoise, thinking the intervention is effective and wanting an RCT undertaken simply to prove this effectiveness to others. This lack of equipoise may be a potential source of tension between the evaluation team and stakeholders who feel ownership of the intervention. Intervention developers may be commercial organizations or local or national policy makers, all of whom can be driven by wider agendas than contributing to the research evidence base. People who have developed the intervention have invested time, money, and reputation in this endeavour, and need to believe in its potential in order to continue with their investment in the future. They may be open to understanding that their intervention could be shown not to work in a full RCT, and open to identifying improvements in the intervention and its implementation during any feasibility study in preparation for the full RCT. Alternatively they may be protective of the content and value of the intervention and resist seeing problems with it or making changes to it. The intervention developers may also have contractual powers over the evaluation team if they have funded the evaluation and the intervention development. Although potentially unwelcome messages for these stakeholders can emerge from different parts of the evaluation, the qualitative research is likely to offer the earliest challenges to these stakeholders.

Moore et al. (2015) discuss the complexity of relationships with these stakeholders in their full report on guidance on process evaluation for complex interventions. They identify the importance of good working relationships with intervention developers because these stakeholder offer insights into the logic model of the intervention and have the power to take action to resolve problems with the intervention. Stakeholders with ownership of the intervention may be required to make changes to the intervention based on qualitative research undertaken at the feasibility stage so that an optimized intervention can be evaluated in the full RCT, or based on qualitative research undertaken alongside the full RCT so that an optimized intervention can be implemented in routine practice post RCT. Moore et al. (2015) recommend agreeing the parameters of these relationships early in the evaluation and continuing to reflect on them throughout the evaluation.

Three types of stakeholders may need specific consideration.

15.2.1 Commercial organizations

Commercial organizations that own interventions present specific potential challenges. They need to consider the financial implications of making changes to their product and may need to obtain board-level approval for any proposed changes. See Box 15.1 for an example of qualitative research being used to identify adaptations to a commercial product prior to use in a pilot RCT. In this example, the time taken to obtain board-level agreement to invest in changing the intervention was much longer than the evaluation team had anticipated. Another example is a feasibility study in preparation for an RCT which considered the need to modify a commercial weight loss intervention

Box 15.1 An example of engaging with commercial stakeholders

A qualitative study to consider the need to adapt existing computerized cognitive behavioural therapy systems for people with multiple sclerosis and depression identified a range of proposed changes to the intervention (Hind et al., 2009). One of these systems was commercial and the team met with the company representative throughout the qualitative research so they were aware of emerging findings and could develop timely action plans for changing the intervention. The intention had been to make changes to the intervention in a six-month period after the qualitative research, and then undertake a pilot RCT of the adapted system. The timetable was unrealistic for the commercial operator and the pilot RCT was undertaken on the original intervention (Cooper et al., 2011). After discussions with their board, and consideration of the cost implications, the commercial operator decided to make many of the changes proposed by the research team but widened the focus of these changes to people with any chronic physical condition and depression rather than the specific condition of multiple sclerosis because this made more sense commercially.

Source: data from Cooper, C.L., et al. (2011). 'Computerised cognitive behavioural therapy for the treatment of depression in people with multiple sclerosis: external pilot trial'. *Trials*, Issue 12, p. 259. © 2011 Cooper et al.

for people with learning disabilities. Here, the commercial organization was part of the research team and wanted to be clear about the credibility of the qualitative research findings prior to committing to making changes to their product. They agreed to make some but not all of the proposed changes because they wanted to test out some changes on a small scale before involving all their franchise holders (Croot et al. submitted). Qualitative researchers may need to be aware of the wider issues affecting any commercial stakeholders and spend time communicating with them about the different perspectives held by academic researchers and commercial organizations so that both parties gain a better understanding of the other's world. This may help both parties to benefit from the relationship within mutually suitable timescales.

15.2.2 National and local policy makers

National or local policy makers may introduce an intervention in a limited number of services or areas for evaluation using a RCT. Qualitative research may identify changes needed to that intervention prior to future roll out across all services or areas. However, some of these changes may be too expensive for policy makers to instigate, or they may not align with wider intentions of the policy makers. In the example in Box 15.1, the qualitative research undertaken prior to a pilot RCT found that people with multiple sclerosis and depression wanted human contact to guide them through the computerized cognitive behavioural therapy. The researchers were aware that local commissioners of the wider service for the general population with depression generally did not fund this aspect of the service due to the cost of providing it (Cooper et al., 2011). This suggested that there would be financial constraints to implementing what might be the optimal intervention for people with multiple sclerosis and depression in the real world. That is, qualitative researchers may need to prioritize any changes they propose to the intervention, and consider their cost implications in the real world.

15.2.3 The evaluation team

The qualitative researchers in a feasibility or full RCT may have been part of the intervention development process. They may be invested in the intervention or have developed tacit knowledge of it. In this case qualitative researchers may need to practise individual reflexivity as they progress through the different stages of evaluation. Early and ongoing 'team reflexivity' may also be needed if the intervention has been developed by other members of the evaluation team. Even where there is no sense of ownership of the intervention within the evaluation team, researchers leading the RCT may not want to hear about major problems with the intervention at the feasibility stage because they are committed to running the full RCT within a specific timeframe. They also may not be keen to hear findings from the qualitative research that appear to criticize how the RCT was run or the intervention delivered within the full RCT. Ongoing team discussions about these issues may help to keep the team open to the insights from the qualitative research and solutions required to address problems with the intervention (see Chapter 14 on teams).

15.3 Governance systems

Governance systems for RCTs may differ by country or funding agency. Funding agencies in the UK require that a trial steering committee is established to provide oversight of the RCT on behalf of the funder. The role of the trial steering committee is to ensure that the RCT is conducted to rigorous standards, with attention to progress, adherence to protocol, patient safety, and new information of relevance to the research question. The data monitoring and ethics committee is a separate body that considers the need for any interim analysis and advises the trial steering committee about the release of any data. Internal governance takes place within clinical trials units, where standard operating procedures are developed to ensure that all procedures are documented and undertaken consistently.

Qualitative researchers need to consider their relationship with these governance systems. Given that data monitoring and ethics committees are interested in the statistical analysis, the qualitative research undertaken alongside a RCT is unlikely to be of relevance to them. However, it is worth considering whether the qualitative research should be overseen by the trial steering committee, and whether it is necessary that it is governed by standard operating procedures. These questions require careful consideration so that qualitative research is neither blindly subsumed within RCT governance processes in a way that leads to a loss of its key strengths, nor excluded from these systems when they could offer importance governance structures for the mixed methods evaluation.

15.3.1 Trial steering committees

One could argue that, whereas RCTs have a specific need for external governance, any qualitative research (and economic modelling) undertaken alongside these RCTs is not of interest to the trial steering committee. A challenge to this argument is that process evaluations can uncover significant adverse events, worrying issues about adherence to a planned intervention (Riley et al., 2005) and affect major decisions about the design of the RCT (Murtagh et al., 2007). It seems sensible to have external governance when issues like this can occur, with decision making on actions taking place in trial steering committees. Over ten years ago Riley et al. (2005) recommended that community intervention trials required a data monitoring committee to debate and make decisions based on emerging findings from the process evaluation. This may happen for some evaluations but it is unlikely to be standard practice. When Cooper et al. (2014) considered how qualitative research should occur within clinical trials units, they identified the problem of researchers independently acting on interim feedback from qualitative research by refining either the intervention or aspects of trial conduct during RCTs. They recommended that clinical trials units explicitly consider how interim reporting of the qualitative research alongside a full RCT should occur and whether the trial steering committee should have access to this information. Potential roles for trial steering committees are summarized in Box 15.2.

The roles and responsibilities of trial steering committees have been reviewed recently (Harman et al., 2015). Indeed qualitative research is being used to help to understand and develop these governance systems: researchers in the

Box 15.2 Potential roles for trial steering committees in relation to qualitative research undertaken with RCTs

- Consideration of proposed changes to the intervention or RCT during full RCTs.
- Oversight of contribution of qualitative research to stopping rules for full RCTs and stop-go criteria if a trial steering committee is established for an external pilot RCT.
- Receipt of the report of the process evaluation prior to the analysis of the RCT data because of the recommendation that this data is analysed prior to knowing the results of the RCT (Moore et al., 2015; Oakley et al., 2006).
- An analysis plan of any integration between the qualitative research and the RCT. For example, if the qualitative research undertaken alongside the RCT generates hypotheses to be tested using the RCT data then the Trials Steering Committee should receive and assess this prior to any analysis occurring (see Chapter 11 on integration).

UK have undertaken non-participant observation of trial steering committees and interviews with their members to consider how they can best improve the conduct of RCTs (Daykin et al., 2014). In another study, members of the trial steering committees and data monitoring and ethics committees have been included in qualitative interviews to explore the conduct of RCTs in a specific field of inquiry (Snowden et al., 2014). This qualitative research reflecting on the practice of these groups may lead to changes in the way they operate in the future. This is an example of how qualitative research is being used to shape how RCTs are conducted more generally. A key action for the future is that both funders and trial steering committee chairs consider the role of this governance system in relation to qualitative research.

15.3.2 Standard operating procedures

A standard operating procedure has been developed for qualitative methods undertaken within a clinical trials unit. It defines good practice, for example that qualitative researchers should contribute from the beginning of the study, and that the main study publication should report on the qualitative component (Rapport et al., 2013). The group that developed this standard operating procedure viewed it as a way of legitimizing qualitative research undertaken in this context, so that it was integrated with the RCT and not treated as an add-on. They explicitly paid attention to maintaining the flexibility of qualitative research within the standard operating procedure.

Each mixed methods evaluation may require its own specific standard operating procedures for the qualitative research because of issues raised by Cooper et al. (2014) where the best approach may be dependent on the design of the RCT. There may be a need to specify how to approach participants for informed consent in the qualitative research, how to maintain confidentiality of participants in the qualitative research, and when to communicate the findings of the qualitative research for a specific study.

15.4 Ethics committees/institutional review boards and attention to ethical issues

The ethical issues facing qualitative research undertaken with RCTs are similar to any qualitative research in terms of the need to obtain ethics committee/institutional review board approval and gain informed consent from research participants. Qualitative researchers will need to consider who they can and cannot approach for participation, the best timing of the qualitative data collection for both the patient and the research, and any research burden given that participants are already participating in an RCT. Participants in RCTs may be very ill or vulnerable and researchers will need consider this when designing the qualitative research.

Members of ethics committees/institutional review boards may have concerns about researchers approaching people who have declined to participate in an RCT or withdrawn from the intervention or RCT. It is essential to be sensitive to people's wishes, but in practice some of these groups of patients are happy to participate in qualitative research, and their participation has raised important issues about problems with the RCT or the intervention (O'Cathain et al., 2016).

When undertaking qualitative research alongside an RCT, researchers often apply for ethics approval for the whole mixed methods evaluation in a single application. Substantial amendments are required for any change to protocol, including amendments to any documentation for participants. This may be challenging for qualitative research where it is good practice for the topic guide to iterate over time. Fortunately, ethics committees often have qualitative research experts on them who understand the need to have evolving topic guides without the need for approval for substantial amendments.

15.5 **Patient and public involvement with research**

In many countries in the world it is considered good practice to have patients and members of the public involved in health research. In the UK this is known as patient and public involvement or PPI (http://www.invo.org.uk/). In the USA this is promoted by the Patient-Centered Outcome Research Institute or PCORI (Frank et al., 2014). Members can contribute to all stages of research, from prioritizing the research question through to dissemination of findings. Researchers are beginning to reflect on how patient and public involvement can best occur within RCTs, with one clinical trials unit creating a standard operating procedure that includes patient and public involvement representatives being members of the trial management group and trial steering committee (Evans et al., 2013). The relationship between the qualitative research and patient and public involvement may need particular consideration because of a lack of clarity about the interface between the two (Hoddinott et al., submitted).

15.5.1 **It may be tempting to label qualitative research as patient and public involvement**

This is not recommended because patient and public involvement members are active decision makers on the study team, shaping and challenging the study. Research participants tend to be passive subjects, offering their views so that researchers can decide how best to act upon them.

15.5.2 **It may be tempting to use patient and public involvement instead of qualitative research**

The views of patient and public involvement members may be sought informally or in a more structured way in discussion groups. Researchers sometimes wrongly label this as focus groups as if it is formal data collection with informed consent. Patient and public involvement members may be asked to comment on the intervention as it is being developed or modified in preparation for the full RCT. If this is the only source of patients' views of the intervention prior to RCT, it is unlikely that it will offer the diversity of sample that can identify the range of problems with complex interventions that may need to be addressed before use in a full RCT. That is, qualitative research is likely to be necessary in conjunction with patient and public involvement.

15.5.3 **Patient and public involvement and qualitative research are undertaken separately**

It is common currently to have both patient and public involvement and qualitative research as separate endeavours within a study. This occurred in the

Healthlines Study which included the development of a telehealth intervention for chronic conditions and its evaluation in two RCTs with embedded qualitative research and economic evaluations (Thomas et al., 2014). Two patient and public involvement representatives were members of the study management group and commented on the intervention as it was developed, the study documentation, preliminary findings of the qualitative research, and interpretation of the overall study findings. The qualitative research was undertaken by academic researchers who interviewed staff and patients receiving the telehealth intervention, and analysed these data before obtaining the views of the wider evaluation team—which included patient and public involvement members—on interpretation.

15.5.4 Patient and public involvement and qualitative research are combined

A recent addition to the knowledge base describes how combining patient and public involvement and qualitative research in the context of a study to inform an RCT ensured the inclusion of 'harder-to-reach' groups than could be achieved through patient and public involvement or qualitative research alone (Morgan et al., 2016). The intervention to be evaluated in the future RCT was to be aimed at women in deprived communities. Existing groups of women from these communities were approached to offer patient and public involvement. In addition their views of the intervention were collected as qualitative data along with those of interviewees sampled in more traditional ways. Their views were different from those of the other interviewees and they were able to identify types of interviewees not already included in the qualitative sample so that a more diverse set of interviews were completed. The research group took a thoughtful approach to this endeavour, tailored to the context of their intervention.

15.6 Key points

- Early and ongoing discussions may be necessary with intervention developers to help the process of relevant groups taking action on the findings of the qualitative research.
- The evaluation team may need to consider the financial implications of proposed changes to the intervention, its implementation, or the RCT based on any qualitative research. Prioritization of proposed changes is likely to be necessary.
- Trial steering committees have important roles to play for oversight of qualitative research findings and actions taken in response to qualitative research findings.

- Standard operating procedures for qualitative research, which attend to the need for a flexible approach to qualitative research, may be a useful addition to clinical trials units.
- Patient and public involvement and qualitative research each make important contributions to RCTs.

15.7 Questions to help you think about your study

- Have you discussed with your wider team how to handle findings emerging from the qualitative research in the context of a lack of equipoise from you, wider team members, intervention developers, or funders?
- Will the trial steering committee receive information about the qualitative research? If so, what specific roles will you want them to deliver?
- If working with a clinical trials unit, do you want the qualitative research to have a standard operating procedure? If so, how will it differ from the one presented by Rapport et al., 2013?
- How do you want your patient and public involvement members to help with your qualitative research? As well as the usual issues like commenting on information sheets, topic guides, and findings, do you want them to help you to identify your sample? What are your justifications for this? Have you identified the necessary resources for this?

Further reading

Morgan, H., Thomson, G., Crossland, N., Dykes, F., Hoddinott, P. (2016). Combining public and patient involvement with qualitative research to engage 'harder-to-reach' populations: service user groups as co-applicants on a platform study for a trial. *Research Involvement and Engagement*, **2**, 7. doi: 10.1186/s40900-016-0023-1.

Rapport, F., Storey, M., Porter, A., Snooks, H., Jones, K., Peconi, J., Sánchez, A., Siebert, S., Thorne, K., Clement, C., Russell, I. (2013). Qualitative research within trials: developing a standard operating procedure for a clinical trials unit. *Trials*, **14**(54). doi: 10.1186/1745-6215-14-54.

Chapter 16

Having an impact on health, health care, and health policy

Overview

Read this chapter to learn about facilitating the use of research findings by

- Team members
- Researchers undertaking related research
- Researchers engaged in synthesizing evidence
- Population, patients, service providers, and policy makers

16.1 Introduction

Researchers generate evidence to improve the health and health care of the population and specific patient groups. To do this, research needs to impact on the practice of research team members, other researchers undertaking related research, other researchers engaged in synthesizing evidence, and patients, practitioners, and policy makers who want to make research evidence-informed decisions. In some countries, university-based research is judged partly by the amount of impact it has in the real world. The focus of this chapter is on the final stage of the research: facilitating the use of the findings of the qualitative research undertaken with RCTs by a variety of stakeholders.

16.2 Impact within a research team

Qualitative researchers cannot assume that team members will act on their findings within a specific study. Planning where and how communication should best occur between team members, and working in a way in which the qualitative research is integral to the whole study, can facilitate the wider team taking action from the qualitative research (see Chapter 14). The types of actions team members take may depend on the phase of evaluation.

16.2.1 Feasibility phase

Qualitative research undertaken prior to a full RCT can reduce the amount of uncertainty about the quality of the intervention, the RCT design or conduct, the outcomes being considered, or how the outcomes are measured. For example, qualitative research with clinicians and patients, undertaken at a pre-trial phase, changed the design of the proposed RCT and the primary outcome to be measured (Rooshenas et al., 2015). The researchers were explicit that this was facilitated by the qualitative researchers being core members of the full research team and presenting emerging findings from the qualitative research to that team. Similarly, the outcome measure to be used in a full RCT was changed after qualitative research at the feasibility phase showed that patients struggled to understand the original outcome measure (Farquahar et al., 2010). In another feasibility study, an additional arm was added to the planned full RCT (Bugge et al., 2013).

There are challenges to taking actions during a feasibility study or at the end of the feasibility study when planning the full RCT. Qualitative research can identify a large number of issues that could be addressed. Researchers need to consider the potential solutions for addressing each problem and the importance, feasibility, and cost of making any proposed changes to the intervention, RCT conduct, or outcomes. Bugge et al. (2013) have developed a process for decision making after a feasibility study for an RCT. The process aims to facilitate a systematic approach to identifying and appraising problems and solutions, and making decision making transparent. It also highlights the tension that can exist between decisions that are good for the RCT and those that are good for the real world implementation of the intervention. Bugge et al. (2013) did not use qualitative research in the study in which they developed their process but nevertheless it is a highly relevant approach that could be adapted to include any qualitative research.

16.2.2 Where qualitative research is undertaken alongside a full RCT

When qualitative research is undertaken alongside a full RCT, researchers may identify sub-group analyses for testing in the full RCT data (see Chapter 11). Statisticians on the team will need to be prepared for this possibility and build it into their analysis plan and timetable. They may have concerns about generation of multiple hypotheses and the post hoc nature of these hypotheses. This will require team discussion about timing, workload and credibility of this hypothesis testing.

If the qualitative research is undertaken to explain the RCT results, the team will need to pay attention to the timing of publication of journal articles to consider whether the impact of the study can be increased overall by simultaneous publication of the RCT and the qualitative research so that the RCT article includes in its discussion section why the intervention did or did not work.

The qualitative research can also have an indirect impact on the team by encouraging members to think about evaluation differently. Team members may take this learning on to future studies.

16.3 **Impact on researchers outside the team**

Researchers outside the original team can only learn from the research if it is disseminated. Dissemination can include presentations at academic conferences, seminars, publication in academic journals, and engagement with social media.

Journal articles reporting the qualitative research need to include key learning points from the study so that other researchers can use the findings of the qualitative research undertaken with an RCT to develop or refine further interventions, or design procedures to run future RCTs more efficiently. Other researchers will find it easier to act upon any qualitative research if the authors are clear about the implications of the qualitative research for the intervention used in the RCT, similar bodies of interventions, and the conduct of similar RCTs in similar populations. It is good practice to make key implications clear in the conclusion of the abstract of a journal article to alert readers to the utility of the article (see Chapter 12). Researchers do not always do this (O'Cathain et al., 2014b), risking loss of learning for research and health care communities.

As discussed in Section 13.5 in Chapter 13, other researchers may consider including qualitative research undertaken with RCTs within systematic reviews. To facilitate this, researchers need to be clear in the abstract of their journal articles that their qualitative research was undertaken in the context of an RCT.

16.4 **Impact in the real world—population, patients, service providers, and policy makers**

Members of the general population, patients, practitioners, or policy makers may wish to implement any effective intervention in a way that attains at least a similar size of effect found in the RCT. Or they may wish to stop using an intervention that has been found to not to be effective. The qualitative research can help them to make decisions by describing the context in which the RCT was undertaken, allowing them to consider the transferability of the RCT results to their own situation; or by describing the intervention as it is practised in the RCT to help them to replicate the intervention and its key mechanisms; or by identifying problems with implementation in the full RCT that can be addressed in future use of the intervention. To facilitate this, researchers need to think about communicating with these stakeholders in meaningful ways. Members of public and patient involvement groups can facilitate dissemination of qualitative research findings to patient groups and the general population by writing easy to read summaries. They can also help researchers to understand the relevance of the research to patients and guide the content of any dissemination.

The chance of having an impact may be increased if researchers work with the relevant health professionals and managers who deliver health care in different health systems internationally, and professional bodies and policy makers within these health systems, to determine the research question for the evaluation in the first place. This can ensure that the research is seen as relevant by these stakeholders before it is undertaken. This applies to both the qualitative research and the RCT. Engaging these stakeholders throughout the research may increase their investment in the results and help them to take appropriate actions in response to the research.

16.5 **Accumulation of knowledge**

Although researchers can think about the impact of individual components of a mixed methods evaluation, it is also useful to consider how the accumulation of knowledge across a number of phases of a study generates impact. Returning to the example in Box 1.1 in Chapter 1, qualitative research identified the problems with an existing service in the first phase of a long study trajectory. This phase led to the design of a more patient-centred service which was then instigated and evaluated using RCTs before being rolled out in different countries where it reduced mortality. Using qualitative research to understand the problems facing patients lay at the foundation of this endeavour and, one could argue, ultimately set it off in the right direction for success.

Stakeholders may not take action from a single study but wait for evidence to be brought together within systematic reviews. These systematic reviews may then be actioned within national guidelines for health care. Traditionally guidelines are based on the results of RCTs but can be expanded to consider the findings from the qualitative research undertaken with these RCTs.

16.6 **The importance of context to impact**

A large review of reviews exploring the barriers and facilitators to the implementation of evidence into practice in primary care identified that the fit between the intervention and the context was critical to the success of implementing the evidence (Lau et al., 2016). This meta-review concluded that health care professionals and policy makers should consider the range of relevant contextual factors, and the dynamic nature of context, to maximize the uptake of complex interventions in primary care. This requires that research studies explicitly consider context. The importance of context within an evaluation and subsequent implementation of complex interventions has been highlighted (Moore et al., 2015; May et al., 2016). Qualitative research can describe context and help stakeholders to understand the role of context in the effectiveness or not of an intervention within both RCTs and routine practice (Raine et al., 2016). That is, qualitative research can be key to the implementation of evidence of effectiveness in the real world.

16.7 Key points

- Qualitative research can have impact by helping fellow team members to address problems with the intervention and RCT conduct before the full expensive evaluation.
- Clear communication of the implications of the qualitative research for the intervention, its implementation or the RCT processes in the abstract of any journal article can facilitate impact.
- Qualitative research early in the trajectory of an evaluation has the potential to set the intervention on the path to success.
- Qualitative research can help a wide variety of stakeholders to understand the role of context on effectiveness and therefore help them to make decisions about using evidence of effectiveness from RCTs.

16.8 Questions to help you think about your study

- Who do you want to listen to your qualitative findings?
- When do you want them to take action on your findings?
- How will you communicate your findings so that each stakeholder knows what action to take and why?
- Have you paid enough attention to context in your qualitative research data collection, analysis and reporting?

Further reading

Lau, R., Stevenson, F., Ong, B.N., Dziedzic, K., Treweek, S., Eldridge, S., Everitt, H., Kennedy, A., Qureshi, N., Rogers, A., Peacock, R., Murray, E. (2016). Achieving change in primary care—causes of the evidence to practice gap: systematic reviews of reviews. *Implementation Science*, **11**(40), doi: 10.1186/s13012-016-0396-4.

References

Abetz, L., Rofail, D., Mertzanis, P., Heelis, R., Rosa, K., Tellefsen, C., Roborel de Climens, A., McBurney, C., Thomas, S. (2009). Alzheimer's disease treatment: assessing caregiver preferences for mode of treatment delivery. *Advances in Therapy*, **26**(6), pp. 627–644. doi: 10.1007/s12325-009-0034-5.

Aoun, S., Deas, K., Toye, C., Ewing, G., Grande, G., Stajduhar, K. (2015). Supporting family caregivers to identify their own needs in end-of-life care: Qualitative findings from a stepped wedge cluster trial. *Palliative Medicine*, **29**(6), pp. 508–517. doi: 10.1177/0269216314566061.

Atkins S., Odendaal, W., Leon, N., Lutge, E., Lewin, S. (2015). Qualitative process evaluation for complex interventions. In: Richards, D.A., Hallberg, I.R. (eds), *Complex interventions in health. An overview of research methods*. London and New York: Routledge, pp. 239–248.

Audrey, S., Holliday, J., Parry-Langdon, N., Campbell, R. (2006). Meeting the challenges of implementing process evaluation within randomized controlled trials: the example of ASSIST (A Stop Smoking in Schools Trial). *Health Education Research*, **21**(3), pp. 366–377. doi: 10.1093/her/cyl029.

Balcazar, H., Rosenthal, L., De Heer, H., Aguirre, M., Flores, L., Vasquez, E., Duarte, M., Schulz, L. (2009). Use of community-based participatory research to disseminate baseline results from a cardiovascular disease randomized community trial for Mexican Americans living in a U.S.-Mexico border community. *Education for Health*, **22**(3), p. 279.

Barbour, R.S. (1999). The case for combining qualitative and quantitative approaches in health services research. *Journal of Health Services Research & Policy*, **4**(1), pp. 39–43.

Barbour, R.S. (2000). The role of qualitative research in broadening the 'evidence base' for clinical practice. *Journal of Evaluation in Clinical Practice*, **6**(2), pp. 155–163. doi: 10.1046/j.1365-2753.2000.00213.x

Bazeley, P. (2009). Analysing mixed methods data. In: Andrew, S. & Halcomb, E.J. (eds) *Mixed methods research for nursing and the health sciences*. Oxford: Wiley-Blackwell, pp. 84–118.

Beal, C.C., Stuifbergen, A., Volker, D., Becker, H. (2009). Women's experiences as members of attention control and experimental intervention groups in a randomized controlled trial. *Canadian Journal of Nursing Research*, **41**(4), pp. 16–31.

Beard, E., Lewis, J.J., Copas, A., Davey, C., Osrin, D., Baio, G., Thompson, J.A., Fielding, K.L., Omar, R.Z., Ononge, S., Hargreaves, J., Prost, A. (2015). Stepped wedge randomised controlled trials: systematic review of studies published between 2010 and 2014. *Trials*, **16**, 353. doi: 10.1186/s13063-015-0839-2.

Behets, F.M., Van Damme, K., Turner, A.N., Rabenja, N.L., Ravelomanana, N.L., Raharinivo, M.S., Zeller, K.A., Rennie, S.M., Swezey, T.A. (2008). Evidence-based planning of a randomized controlled trial on diaphragm use for prevention of sexually transmitted infections. *Sexually Transmitted Diseases*, **35**, pp. 238–242. doi: 10.1097/OLQ.0b013e31815abaa2.

BioMed Central (2017). *Pilot and feasibility studies*. https://pilotfeasibilitystudies.biomedcentral.com, accessed 24/2/17.

Bonell, C., Fletcher, A., Morton, M., Lorenc, T., Moore, L. (2012). Realist randomised controlled trials: a new approach to evaluating complex public health interventions. *Social Science & Medicine*, **75**(12), pp. 2299–2306. doi: 10.1016/j.socscimed.2012.08.032.

Bonell, C., Jamal, F., Melendez-Torres, G.J., et al. (2014). 'Dark logic': theorising the harmful consequences of public health interventions. *Journal of Epidemiology and Community Health*, **69**, pp. 95–98.

Bosch, M., Tavender, E.J., Brennan, S.E., Knott, J., Gruen, R.L., Green, S.E. (2016). The many organisational factors relevant to planning change in emergency care departments: a qualitative study to inform a cluster randomised controlled trial aiming to improve the management of patients with mild traumatic brain injuries. *PLoS ONE*, **11**(2), e0148091. doi:10.1371/journal.pone.0148091

Braun, V., Clarke, V. (2006). Using thematic analysis in psychology. *Qualitative Research in Psychology*, **3**, pp. 77–101. doi: 10.1191/1478088706qp063oa.

Brookes, S., Biddle, L., Paterson, C., Woolhead, G., Dieppe, P. (2007). 'Me's me and you's you': exploring patients' perspectives of single patient (n-of-1) trials in the UK. *Trials*, **8**, 10. doi: 10.1186/1745-6215-8-10.

Bryman, A. (2012). *Social Research Methods* (4th ed.). Oxford: OUP.

Bryman, A. (1988). *Quantity and Quality in Social Research (Contemporary Social Research)*. Abingdon: Routledge.

Bugge, C., Williams, B., Hagen, S., Logan, J., Glazener, C., Pringle, S., Sinclair, L. (2013). A process for Decision-making after Pilot and feasibility Trials (ADePT): development following a feasibility study of a complex intervention for pelvic organ prolapse. *Trials*, **14**, 353. doi: 10.1186/1745-6215-14-353.

Campbell, N.C., Murray, E., Darbyshire, J., Emery, J., Farmer, A., Griffiths, F., Guthrie, B., Lester, H., Wilson, P., Kinmonth, A.L. (2007). Designing and evaluating complex interventions to improve health care. *BMJ*, **334**(7591), pp. 455–459. doi: 10.1136/bmj.39108.379965.BE.

Campbell, M., Fitzpatrick, R., Haines, A., Kinmonth, A.L., Sandercock, P., Spiegelhalter, D., Tyrer, P. (2000). *Framework for design and evaluation of complex interventions to improve health*. BMJ, **321**(7262), pp. 694–696.

Campbell, R., Quilty, B., Dieppe, P. (2003). Discrepancies between patients' assessments of outcome: qualitative study nested within a randomised controlled trial. *BMJ*, **326**, pp. 252–253. doi: 10.1136/bmj.326.7383.252.

Campbell, R., Rawlins, E., Wells, S., Kipping, R.R., Chittleborough, C.R., Peters, T.J., Lawlor, D.A., Jago, R. (2015). Intervention fidelity in a school-based diet and physical activity intervention in the UK: Active for Life Year 5. *International Journal of Behavioral Nutrition and Physical Activity*, **12**, 141. doi: 10.1186/s12966-015-0300-7.

Cane, J., O'Connor, D., Michie, S. (2012). Validation of the theoretical domains framework for use in behaviour change and implementation research. *Implementation Science*, **7**, p. 37. doi: 10.1186/1748-5908-7-37.

CFHealthHub. (2016). CFHealthHub: development and evaluation of an intervention to support adherence to treatment in adults with cystic fibrosis. www.sheffield.ac.uk/scharr/sections/dts/ctru/cfhealthhub, accessed 24/2/17

Connelly, L.M., Yoder, L.H. (2000). Improving qualitative proposals: common problem areas. *Clinical Nurse Specialist*, **14**(2), pp. 69–74. doi: 10.1097/00002800-200003000-00009.

Cooper, C.L., Hind, D., Parry, G.D., Isaac, C.L., Dimairo, M., O'Cathain, A., Rose, A., Freeman, J.V., Martin, L., Kaltenthaler, E., Thake, A., Sharrack, B. (2011). Computerised cognitive behavioural therapy for the treatment of depression in people with multiple sclerosis: external pilot trial. *Trials*, **12**, p. 259. doi: 10.1186/1745-6215-12-259.

Cooper, C.L., O'Cathain, A., Hind, D., Adamson, J., Lawton, J., Baird, W. (2014). Conducting qualitative research within clinical trials units: avoiding potential pitfalls. *Contemporary Clinical Trials*, **38**, pp. 338–343. doi: 10.1016/j.cct.2014.06.002.

Coupe, N., Anderson, E., Gask, L., Sykes, P., Richards, D.A., Chew-Graham, C. (2014). Facilitating professional liaison in collaborative care for depression in UK primary care; a qualitative study utilising normalisation process theory. *BMC Family Practice*, 2014, 15, p. 78. doi: 10.1186/1471-2296-15-78.

Craig, P., Dieppe, P., Macintyre, S., Michie, S., Nazareth, I., Petticrew, M. (2008). Developing and evaluating complex interventions: the new Medical Research Council guidance. *BMJ*, **337**, a1655. doi: 10.1136/bmj.a1655.

Creswell, J.W. (2002). *Research design: qualitative, quantitative, and mixed methods approaches*. Thousand Oaks, CA: Sage Publications.

Creswell, J., Plano Clark, V. (2007). *Designing and Conducting Mixed Methods Research*. Thousand Oaks, CA: Sage Publications.

Creswell, J.W., Fetters, M.D., Plano Clark, V.L., Morales, A. (2009). Mixed methods intervention trials. In: Andrew, S., Halcomb, E.J. (eds). *Mixed methods research for nursing and the health sciences*. Oxford: Wiley-Blackwell, pp. 161–180.

Creswell, J.W., Klassen, A.C., Plano Clark, V.L., Smith, K.C., Office of Behavioral and Social Sciences Research (OBSSR). (2011). *Best practices for mixed methods research in the health sciences*. Bethesda, MD: National Institutes of Health.

Creswell, J.W., Plano Clark, V.L. (2011). *Designing and Conducting Mixed Methods Research* (2nd edn). Thousand Oaks, CA: Sage Publications.

Croot, L., Rimmer, M., Salway, S., Hatton, C., Dowse, E., Lavin, J., Bennett, S.E., Harris, J., O'Cathain, A. Adjusting a mainstream weight management intervention for people with intellectual disabilities: a user centred approach, submitted.

Curran, J.A., Brehaut, J., Patey, A.M., Osmond, M., Stiell, I., Grimshaw, J.M. (2013). Understanding the Canadian adult CT head rule trial: use of the theoretical domains frameworks for process evaluation. *Implementation Science*, **8**, p. 25. doi: 10.1186/1748-5908-8-25.

Curry, L.A., O'Cathain, A., Plano Clark, V.L., Aroni, R., Fetters, M., Berg, D. (2012). The role of group dynamics in mixed methods health sciences research teams. *Journal of Mixed Methods Research*, **6**(1), pp. 5–20. doi: 10.1177/1558689811416941.

Curry, L., Nunez-Smith, M. (2015). *Mixed methods in health sciences research: a practical primer*. Thousand Oaks, CA: Sage Publications.

Davidoff, F., Dixon-Woods, M., Leviton, L., Michie, S. (2015). Demystifying theory and its use in improvement. *BMJ Quality and Safety*, **24**(3), pp. 228–238. doi: 10.1136/bmjqs-2014-003627.

Daykin, A.R., Heawood, A., Lane, A., Macefield, R., McCann, S., Gamble, C., Shorter, G. (2014). A qualitative study of group decision making and member roles to understand and improve how trial oversight committees contribute to trial conduct. Society for Clinical Trials Annual Meeting (abstract). doi: 10.1186/1745-6215-16-S2-P78.

Dimairo, M., Boote, J., Julious, S.A., Nicholl, J.P., Todd, S. (2015). Missing steps in a staircase: a qualitative study of the perspectives of key stakeholders on the use of adaptive designs in confirmatory trials. *Trials*, **16**, 430. doi: 10.1186/s13063-015-0958-9.

Donovan, J.L., Mills, N., Smith, M., Brindle, L., Jacoby, A., Peters, T., Frankel, S., Neal, D., Hamdy, F. (2002). Quality improvement report: improving design and conduct of randomised trials by embedding them in qualitative research: ProtecT (prostate testing for cancer and treatment) study. Commentary: presenting unbiased information to patients can be difficult. *BMJ*, **325**(7367), pp. 766–770. doi: 10.1136/bmj.325.7367.766.

Donovan, J.L., Rooshenas, L., Jepson, M., Elliott, D., Wade, J., Avery, K., Mills, N., Wilson, C., Paramasivan, S., Blazeby J. (2016). Optimising recruitment and informed consent in randomised controlled trials: the development and implementation of the Quintet Recruitment Intervention (QRI), *Trials*, **17**(1), p. 283. doi: 10.1186/s13063-016-1391-4.

Drabble, S.J., O'Cathain, A., Thomas, K.J., Rudolph, A., Hewison, J. (2014). Describing qualitative research undertaken with randomised controlled trials in grant proposals: a documentary analysis. *BMC Medical Research Methodology*, pp. 14–24. doi: 10.1186/1471-2288-14-24.

Drabble, S.J., O'Cathain, A. (2015). Moving from randomised controlled trials to mixed methods intervention evaluations. In: Hesse-Biber, S., Johnson, B. (eds.). *The Oxford handbook of multimethod and mixed methods research inquiry*. Oxford University Press. pp. 406–425.

Duan, N., Kravitz, R. L., Schmid, C. H. (2013). Single patient (n-of-1) trials: a pragmatic clinical decision methodology for patient-centered comparative effectiveness research. *Journal of Clinical Epidemiology*, **66**, S1–S28. doi: 10.1016/j.jclinepi.2013.04.006.

Eldridge, S.M., Lancaster, G.A., Campbell, M.J., Thabane, L., Hopewell, S., Coleman, C.L., Bond, C.M. (2016). Defining feasibility and pilot studies in preparation for randomised controlled trials: development of a conceptual framework. *PLoS ONE 11*, 3, e0150205. doi: 10.1371/journal.pone.0150205.

Ellard, D.R., Taylor, S.J., Parsons, S., Thorogood, M. (2011). The OPERA trial: a protocol for the process evaluation of a randomised trial of an exercise intervention for older people in residential and nursing accommodation. *Trials*, **12**, 28. doi: 10.1186/1745-6215-12-28.

Emsley, R., Dunn, G., White, I.R. (2010). Mediation and moderation of treatment effects in randomised controlled trials of complex interventions. *Statistical Methods in Medical Research*, **19**(3), pp. 237–270. doi: 10.1177/0962280209105014.

Evans, B.A., Bedson, E., Bell, P., Hutchings, H., Lowes, L., Rea, D., Seagrove, A., Siebert, S., Smith, G., Snooks, H., Thomas, M., Thorne, K., Russell, I., WWORTH. (2013). Involving service users in trials: developing a standard operating procedure. *Trials*, **14**, 219. doi: 10.1186/1745-6215-14-219.

Fàbregues, S., Molina-Azorín, J.F. (2016). Addressing quality in mixed methods research: A review and recommendations for a future agenda. *Quality & Quantity*, pp. 1–17. doi: 10.1007/s11135-016-0449-4.

Farmer, T., Robinson, K., Elliott, S.J., Eyles, J. (2006). Developing and implementing a triangulation protocol for qualitative health research. *Qualitative Health Research*, **16**, pp. 377–394. doi: 10.1177/1049732305285708

Farquhar, M., Ewing, G., Higginson, I.J., Booth, S. (2010). The experience of using the SEIQoL-DW with patients with advanced chronic obstructive pulmonary disease (COPD): issues of process and outcome. *Quality of Life Research*, **19** (5), pp. 619–629. doi: 10.1007/s11136-010-9631-7.

Fetters, M.D., Curry, L.A., Creswell, J.W. (2013). Achieving integration in mixed methods designs—principles and practices. *Health Services Research*, **48**(6, pt. 2), pp. 2134–2156. doi: 10.1111/1475-6773.12117.

Fielding, N., Fielding, J. (1986). *Linking data (qualitative research methods)*. Thousand Oaks, CA: Sage Publications.

Flemming, K., Adamson, J., Atkin, K. (2008). Improving the effectiveness of interventions in palliative care: the potential role of qualitative research in enhancing evidence from randomized controlled trials. *Palliative Medicine*, **22**, pp. 123–131. doi: 10.1177/0269216307087319.

Frank, L., Basch, E., Selby J.V., Patient-Centered Outcomes Research Institute. (2014). The PCORI perspective on patient-centered outcomes research. *Journal of the American Medical Association*. **312** (15), pp. 1513–1514. doi: 10.1001/jama.2014.11100.

Garcia, J., Colson, P.W., Parker, C., Hirsch, J.S. (2015). Passing the baton: community-based ethnography to design a randomized clinical trial on the effectiveness of oral pre-exposure prophylaxis for HIV prevention among black men who have sex with men. *Contemporary Clinical Trials*, **45**(Part B), pp. 244–251. doi: 10.1016/j.cct.2015.10.005.

Giddings, L.S. (2006). Mixed-methods research Positivism dressed in drag? *Journal of Research in Nursing*, **11**(3), pp. 195–203. doi: 10.1177/1744987106064635.

Glasgow, R.E., Vogt, T.M., Boles, S.M. (1999). Evaluating the public health impact of health promotion interventions: the RE-AIM framework. *American Journal of Public Health*, **89**(9), pp. 1322–1327.

Glenton, C., Lewin, S., Scheel, I.B. (2011). Still too little qualitative research to shed light on results from reviews of effectiveness trials: a case study of a Cochrane review on the use of lay health workers. *Implementation science*, **6**(53), doi: 10.1186/1748-5908-6-53.

Goodkind, J.R., Amer, S., Christian, C., Hess, J.M., Bybee, D., Isakson, B.L., Baca, B., Ndayisenga, M., Greene, R.N., Shantzek, C. (2017). Challenges and innovations in a community-based participatory randomized controlled trial. *Health Education & Behaviour*, **44**(1), pp. 123–130. doi: 10.1177/1090198116639243.

Grant, A., Dreischulte, T., Treweek, S., Guthrie, B. (2012). Study protocol of a mixed-methods evaluation of a cluster randomized trial to improve the safety of NSAID and antiplatelet prescribing: data-driven quality improvement in primary care. *Trials*, **13**, p. 154. doi: 10.1186/1745-6215-13-154.

Grant, A., Treweek, S., Dreischulte, T., Foy, R., Guthrie, B. (2013). Process evaluations for cluster-randomised trials of complex interventions: a proposed framework for design and reporting. *Trials*, **14**, p. 15. doi: 10.1186/1745-6215-14-15.

Greene, J.C., Benjamin, L., Goodyear, L. (2001). The merits of mixing methods in evaluation. *Evaluation*, **7**(1), pp. 25–44. doi: 10.1177/13563890122209504.

Greenhalgh, T., Robert, G., Macfarlane, F., Bate, P., Kyriakidou, O. (2004). Diffusion of innovations in service organizations: systematic review and recommendations. *Milbank Q*. **82**(4), pp. 581–629. doi: 10.1111/j.0887-378X.2004.00325.x

Greenhalgh, T., Annandale, E., Ashcroft, R., Barlow, J., Black, N., Bleakley, A., et al. (2016). An open letter to the BMJ editors on qualitative research. *BMJ*, **352**, p i563. doi: 10.1136/bmj.i563.

Grissmer, D.W. (2016). *A guide to incorporating multiple methods in randomized control trials to assess intervention effects* (2nd edn). http://www.apa.org/ed/schools/teaching-learning/mixed-methods.aspx.

Harman, N.L., Conroy, E.J., Lewis, S.C., Murray, G., Norrie, J., Sydes, M.R., Lane, J.A., Altman, D.G., Baigent, C., Bliss. J.M., Campbell, M.K., Elbourne, D., Evans, S., Sandercock, P., Gamble, C. (2015). Exploring the role and function of trial steering committees: results of an expert panel meeting. *Trials*, **16**, 597. doi: 10.1186/s13063-015-1125-z.

Hawe, P., Shiell, A., Riley, T. (2004). Complex interventions: how far "out of control" should a randomised controlled trial be? *BMJ*, **328**, pp. 1561–1563. doi: 10.1136/bmj.328.7455.1561.

Hesse-Biber, S. (2012). Weaving a multimethodology and mixed methods praxis into randomized control trials to enhance credibility. *Qualitative Inquiry*, **18**(10), pp. 876–889. doi: 10.1177/1077800412456964.

Higginson, I.J., Evans, C.J., Grande, G., Preston, N., Morgan, M., McCrone, P., Lewis, P., Fayers, P., Harding, R., Hotopf, M., Murray, S.A., Benalia, H., Gysels, M., Farquhar, M., Todd, C., MORECare. (2013). Evaluating complex interventions in end of life care: the MORECare Statement on good practice generated by a synthesis of transparent expert consultations and systematic reviews. *BMC Medicine*, **11**, p. 111. doi: 10.1186/1741-7015-11-111.

Hind, D., O'Cathain, A., Cooper, C.L., Parry, G.D., Isasac, C.L., Rose, A., Martin, L., Sharrack, B. (2009). The acceptability of computerised cognitive behaviour therapy for the treatment of depression in people with chronic physical disease: a qualitative study of people with multiple sclerosis. *Psychology and Health*, **25**(6), pp. 699–712. doi: 10.1080/08870440902842739.

Hoddinott, P., Britten, J., Pill, R. (2010). Why do interventions work in some places and not others: a breastfeeding support group trial. *Social Science & Medicine*, **70**(5), pp. 769–778. doi: 10.1016/j.socscimed.2009.10.067.

Hoddinott, P., Craig, L., Maclennan, G., Boyers, D., Vale, L., NHS Grampian and the University of Aberdeen FEST project team. (2012). Process evaluation for the FEeding Support Team (FEST) randomised controlled feasibility trial of proactive and reactive telephone support for breastfeeding women living in disadvantaged areas. *BMJ Open*, **2**(2), e001039, doi: 10.1136/bmjopen-2012-001039.

Hoddinott P, Pollock A, O'Cathain A, Boyer I, Taylor J, MacDonald C, Oliver S, Donovan JL. How to incorporate patient and public perspectives into the design and conduct of research, submitted.

Hsieh, S.F., Shannon, S.E. (2005). Three approaches to qualitative content analysis. *Qualitative Health Research*, **15** (9), pp. 1277–1288. doi: 10.1177/1049732305276687.

Hubbard, G., Adams, R., Campbell, A., Kidd, L., Leslie, S.J., Munro, J., Watson, A. (2016). Is referral of postsurgical colorectal cancer survivors to cardiac rehabilitation feasible and acceptable? A pragmatic pilot randomised controlled trial with embedded qualitative study. *BMJ Open*, **6**, e009284. doi: 10.1136/bmjopen-2015-009284.

Hutchings, H.A., Thorne, K., Jerzembek, G.S., Cheung, W.Y., Cohen, D., Durai, D., Rapport, F.L., Seagrove, A.C., Williams, J.G., Russell, I.T. (2016). Successful development and testing of a Method for Aggregating The Reporting of Interventions in Complex Studies (MATRICS). *Journal of Clinical Epidemiology*, **69**(0), pp. 193–198. doi: 10.1016/j.jclinepi.2015.08.006.

Jack, S.M., Sheehan, D., Gonzalez, A., MacMillan, H.L., Catherine, N., Waddell, C., for the BCHCP Process Evaluation Research Team. (2015). British Columbia Healthy Connections Project process evaluation: a mixed methods protocol to describe the implementation and delivery of the Nurse-Family Partnership in Canada. *BMC Nursing*, **14**, p. 47, doi: 10.1186/s12912-015-0097-3.

Jago, R., Rawlins, E., Kipping, R.R., Wells, S., Chittleborough, C., Peters, T.J., Mytton, J., Lawlor, D.A., Campbell, R. (2015). Lessons learned from the AFLY5 RCT process evaluation: implications for the design of physical activity and nutrition interventions in schools. *BMC Public Health*, **15**, p. 946. doi:10.1186/s12889-015-2293-1

Jamal, F., Fletcher, A., Shackleton, N., Elbourne, D., Viner, R., Bonell, C. (2015). The three stages of building and testing midlevel theories in a realist RCT: A theoretical and methodological case-example. *Trials*, **16**, p. 466. doi: 10.1186/s13063-015-0980-y.

Johnson, R.B., Schoonenboom J. (2015). Adding qualitative and mixed methods research to health intervention studies: interacting with differences. *Quality Health Research*, **26**(5), pp. 587–602. doi: 10.1177/1049732315617479.

Keeley, T., Williamson, P., Callery, P., Jones, L.L., Mathers, J., Jones, J., Young, B., Calvert, M. (2016). The use of qualitative methods to inform Delphi surveys in core outcome set development. *Trials*, **17**(1), p. 230. doi: 10.1186/s13063-016-1356-7.

W.K. Kellogg Foundation. (2004) *Logic model development guide. using logic models to bring together planning, evaluation, and action.* https://www.wkkf.org/resource-directory/resource/2006/02/wk-kellogg-foundation-logic-model-development-guide, accessed 20/11/17

Khan, M.A., Walley, J., Newell, J., Imdad, N. (2000). Tuberculosis in Pakistan: sSocio-cultural constraints and opportunities in treatment. *Social Science & Medicine*, **50**(2), pp. 247–254. doi: 10.1016/S0277-9536(99)00279-8.

Kipping, R., Payne, C., Lawlor, D.A. (2008). Randomised controlled trial adapting American school obesity prevention to England. *Archives of Disease in Childhood*, **93**(6), pp. 469–473. doi: 10.1136/adc.2007.116970.

Kipping, R.R., Jago, R., Lawlor, D.A. (2012). Developing parent involvement in a school-based child obesity prevention intervention: a qualitative study and process evaluation. *Journal of Public Health (Oxford)*, **34**(2), pp. 236–44. doi: 10.1093/pubmed/fdr076.

Kipping, R.R., Howe, L.D., Jago, R., Campbell, R., Wells, S., Chittleborough, C.R., Mytton, J., Noble, S.M., Peters, T.J., Lawlor, D.A. (2014). Effect of intervention aimed at increasing physical activity, reducing sedentary behaviour, and increasing fruit and vegetable consumption in children: Active for Life Year 5 (AFLY5) school based cluster randomised controlled trial. *BMJ*, **348**, g3256. doi: 10.1136/bmj.g3256.

Lau, R., Stevenson, F., Ong, B.N., Dziedzic, K., Treweek, S., Eldridge, S., Everitt, H., Kennedy, A., Qureshi, N., Rogers, A., Peacock, R., Murray, E. (2016). Achieving change in primary care—causes of the evidence to practice gap: systematic reviews of reviews. *Implementation Science*, **11**, p. 40, doi: 10.1186/s13012-016-0396-4.

Lawlor, D.A., Jago, R., Noble, S.M., Chittleborough, C.R., Campbell, R., Mytton, J., Howe, L.D., Peters, T.J., Kipping, R.R. (2011). The Active for Life Year 5 (AFLY5) school based cluster randomised controlled trial: Study protocol for a randomized controlled trial. *Trials*, **12**, pp. 181–94. doi: 10.1186/1745-6215-12-181.

Lawlor, D.A., Peters, T., Howe, L., Noble, S., Kipping, R., Jago, R. (2013). The Active for Life Year 5 (AFLY5) school-based cluster randomised controlled trial protocol: detailed statistical analysis plan. *Trials*, **14**, 234. doi: 10.1186/1745-6215-14-234.

Lawlor, D.A., Howe, L.D., Anderson, E.L., Kipping, R.R., Campbell, R., Wells, S., Chittleborough, C.R., Peters, T.J., Jago, R. (2016a). The Active for Life Year 5 (AFLY5) school-based cluster randomised controlled trial: effect on potential mediators. *BMC Public Health*, **16**, 68. doi: 10.1186/s12889-016-2734-5.

Lawlor, D.A., Kipping, R.R., Anderson, E.L., Howe, L.D., Chittleborough, C.R., Moure-Fernandez, A., Noble, S.M., Rawlins, E., Wells, S.L., Peters, T.J., Jago, R., Campell, R. (2016b). Active for Life Year 5: a cluster randomised controlled trial of a primary school-based intervention to increase levels of physical activity, decrease sedentary behaviour and improve diet. *Public Health Research*, **4**, p. 7.

Lawton, J., Kirkham, J., White, D., Rankin, D., Cooper, C., Heller, S. (2015). Uncovering the emotional aspects of working on a clinical trial: a qualitative study of the experiences and views of staff involved in a type 1 diabetes trial. *Trials*, **16**, 3. doi: 10.1186/1745-6215-16-3.

Lewin, S., Glenton, C., and **Oxman, A.D.** (2009). Use of qualitative methods alongside randomised controlled trials of complex healthcare interventions: Methodological study. *British Medical Journal*, **339**, b3496. doi: 10.1136/bmj.b3496.

Lewin, S., Glenton, C., Munthe-Kaas, H., Carlsen, B., Colvin, C.J., Gülmezoglu, M., et al. (2015). Using qualitative evidence in decision making for health and social interventions: an approach to assess confidence in findings from qualitative evidence syntheses (GRADE-CERQual). *PLoS Med*, **12**(10), e1001895. doi: 10.1371/journal.pmed.1002065.

Leykum, L.K., Pugh, J.A., Lanham, H.J., Harmon, J., McDaniel, R.R. Jr. (2009). Implementation research design: integrating participatory action research into randomized controlled trials. *Implementation Science*, **4**, p. 69. doi: 10.1186/1748-5908-4-69.

Linnan, L., Steckler, A. (2002). Process evaluations for public health interventions and research. In Steckler, A. & Linnan, L., (eds). *Process evaluations for public health interventions and research*. San Francisco, CA: Jossey-Bass, pp. 1–23.

Liu, H., Lindley, R., Alim, M., Felix, C., Gandhi, D.B., Verma, S.J., Tugnawat, D.K., Syrigapu, A., Ramamurthy, R.K., Pandian, J.D., Walker, M., Forster, A., Anderson, C.S., Langhorne, P., Murthy, G.V., Shamanna, B.R., Hackett, M.L., Maulik, P.K., Harvey, L.A. (2016). Protocol for process evaluation of a randomised controlled trial of family-led rehabilitation post stroke (ATTEND) in India. *BMJ Open*, **6**(9), e012027. doi: 10.1136/bmjopen-2016-012027.

Loder, E., Groves, T., Schroter, S., Merino, J.G., Weber, W. (2016). Qualitative research and the *BMJ*. *BMJ*, **352**, p. i641. doi: 10.1136/bmj.i641.

Marchal, B., Westhorp, G., Wong, G., Van Belle, S., Greenhalgh, T., Kegels, G., Pawson, R. (2013). Realist RCTs of complex interventions—an oxymoron. *Social Science & Medicine*, **94**, pp. 124–128. doi: 10.1016/j.socscimed.2013.06.025.

Masood, Y., Lovell, K., Lunat, F., Atif, N., Waheed, W., Rahman, A., Mossabir, R., Chaudhry, N., Husain, N. (2015). Group psychological intervention for postnatal depression: a nested qualitative study with British South Asian women. *BMC Womens Health*, **15**, 109. doi: 10.1186/s12905-015-0263-5.

May, C.R., Finch, T., Ballini, L., MacFarlane, A., Mair, F., Murray, E., Treweek, S., Rapley, T. (2011). Evaluating complex interventions and health technologies using normalization process theory: development of a simplified approach and web enabled toolkit. *BMC Health Services Research*, **11**, p. 245. doi: 10.1186/1472-6963-11-245.

May, C.R., Johnson, M., and **Finch, T.** (2016). Implementation, context and complexity. *Implementation Science*, **11**, p. 141. doi: 10.1186/s13012-016-0506-3.

Mays, N. and **Pope C.** (2000). Qualitative research in health care: Assessing quality in qualitative research. *BMJ*, **320**(7226), pp. 50–52. doi: 10.1136/bmj.320.7226.50.

McCambridge, J., Witton, J., Elbourne, D.R. (2014). Systematic review of the Hawthorne effect: new concepts are needed to study research participation effects. *Journal of Clinical Epidemiology*, **67**(3), pp. 267–277. doi: 10.1016/j.jclinepi.2013.08.015.

McEvoy, R., Ballini, L., Maltoni, S., O'Donnell, C.A., Mair, F.S., Macfarlane, A. (2014). A qualitative systematic review of studies using the normalization process theory to research implementation processes. *Implementation Science*, **9**, p. 2. doi: 10.1186/1748-5908-9-2.

McMullen, H., Griffiths, C., Leber, W., Greenhalgh, T. (2015). Explaining high and low performers in complex intervention trials: a new model based on diffusion of innovations theory. *Trials*, **16**, p. 242. doi: 10.1186/s13063-015-0755-5.

McQueen A., Bartholomew, L.K., Greisinger, A.J., Medina, G.G., Hawley, S.T., Haidet, P., Bettencourt, J.L., Shokar, N.K., Ling, B.S., Vernon, S.W. (2009). Behind closed doors: physician-patient discussions about colorectal cancer screening. *Journal of General Internal Medicine*, **24**(11), pp. 1228–1235.

Mertens, D.M. and **Tarsilla, M.** (2015). 'Mixed-Methods Evaluation'. In: Hesse-Biber, S.N., Johnson, R.B. (eds) *The Oxford handbook of multimethod and mixed methods research inquiry*. Oxford Library of Psychology. Oxford: Oxford University Press.

Miles, M., Huberman, A. (1994). *Qualitative data analysis: an expanded sourcebook*. Thousand Oaks, CA: Sage Publications.

Moffatt, S., White, M., Mackintosh, J., Howel, D. (2006). Using quantitative and qualitative data in health services research—what happens when mixed method findings conflict? *BMC Health Services Research*, **6**, p. 28. doi: 10.1186/1472-6963-6-28.

Moodie, E.E., Karran, J.C., Shortreed, S.M. (2016). A case study of SMART attributes: a qualitative assessment of generalizability, retention rate, and trial quality. *Trials*, **17**(1), p. 242. doi: 10.1186/s13063-016-1368-3.

Moore, G., Audrey, S., Barker, M., Bond, L., Bonell, C., Cooper, C., Hardeman, W., Moore, L., O'Cathain, A., Tannaze, T., Wight, D., Baird, J. (2015). Process evaluation of complex interventions. Medical Research Council guidance. *BMJ*, **350**, p. h1258. doi: 10.1136/bmj.h1258.

Morgan, D.L. (1998). Practical strategies for combining qualitative and quantitative methods: applications to health research. *Qualitative Health Research*, **8**, p. 362. doi: 10.1177/104973239800800307.

Morgan, D.L. (2007). Paradigms lost and pragmatism regained methodological implications of combining qualitative and quantitative methods. *Journal of Mixed Methods Research*, **1**(1), pp. 48–76. doi: 10.1177/2345678906292462.

Morgan, H., Thomson, G., Crossland, N., Dykes, F., Hoddinott, P. (2016). Combining public and patient involvement with qualitative research to engage 'harder-to-reach' populations: service user groups as co-applicants on a platform study for a trial. *Research Involvement and Engagement*, **2**, p. 7. doi: 10.1186/s40900-016-0023-1.

Moran-Ellis, J., Alexander, V.D., Cronin, A., Dickinson, M., Fielding, J., Sleney, J., Thomas, H. (2006). Triangulation and integration: processes, claims and implications. *Qualitative Research*, **6**, pp. 45–59. doi: 10.1177/1468794106058870.

Morgan-Trimmer, S., Wood, F. (2016). Ethnographic methods for process evaluations of complex health behaviour interventions. *Trials*, **17**, p. 232. doi: 10.1186/s13063-016-1340-2.

Munro, A., Bloor, M. (2010). Process evaluation: The new miracle ingredient in public health research? *Qualitative Research*, **10**, pp. 699–713. doi: 10.1177/1468794110380522.

Murphy, E., Dingwall, R., Greatbatch, D., Parker, S., Watson, P. (1998). Qualitative research methods in health technology assessment: a review of the literature. *Health Technology Assessment*, **2**(16): pp. iii–ix, 1–274. doi: 10.3310/hta2160.

Murray, E., Treweek, S., Pope, C., MacFarlane, A., Ballini, L., Dowrick, C., Finch, T., Kennedy, A., Mair, F., O'Donnell, C., Ong, B.N., Rapley, T., Rogers, A., May, C. (2010). Normalisation process theory: a framework for developing, evaluating and implementing complex interventions. *BMC Medicine*, **8**, p. 63. doi: 10.1186/1741-7015-8-63.

Murtagh, M.J., Thomson, R.G., May, C.R., Rapley, T., Heaven, B.R., Graham, R.H., Kaner, E.F., Stobbart, L., Eccles, M.P. (2007). Qualitative methods in a randomised controlled trial: the role of an integrated qualitative process evaluation in providing evidence to discontinue the intervention in one arm of a trial of a decision support tool. *Quality &Safety in Health Care*, **16**, pp. 224–229. doi: 10.1136/qshc.2006.018499.

Nakash, R.A., Hutton, J.L., Lamb, S.E., Gates, S., Fisher, J. (2008). Response and non-response to postal questionnaire follow-up in a clinical trial—a qualitative study of the patient's perspective. *Journal of Evaluation in Clinical Practice*, **14**(2), pp. 226–235. doi: 10.1111/j.1365-2753.2007.00838.x.

Noyes, J., Popay, J., Pearson, A., Hannes K., Booth, A., **on behalf of the Cochrane Qualitative Research Methods Group**. (2011). Qualitative research and Cochrane reviews. In: Higgins, J.P.T., Green, S. (eds). *Cochrane handbook for systematic reviews of interventions* Version 5.1.0 [updated March 2011]. The Cochrane Collaboration, 2011. www.handbook.cochrane.org.

Oakley, A., Strange, V., Bonell, C., Allen, E., Stephenson, J. (2006). Process evaluation in randomised controlled trials of complex interventions. *BMJ*, **332**, 413. doi: 10.1136/bmj.332.7538.413.

O'Cathain, A., Walters, S.J., Nicholl, J.P., Thomas, K.J., Kirkham, M. (2002). Use of evidence based leaflets to promote informed choice in maternity care: randomised controlled trial in everyday practice. *BMJ*, **324**, pp. 643–646.

O'Cathain, A., Murphy, E., Nicholl, J.P. (2008). The quality of mixed methods studies in health services research. *Journal of Health Services Research and Policy*, **13**(2), pp. 92–98. doi: 10.1258/jhsrp.2007.007074.

O'Cathain, A. (2009), Reporting results. In: Andrew, S., Halcomb, E. (eds). *Mixed methods research for nursing and the health sciences*. Oxford: Blackwell Publishing, pp. 135–158.

O'Cathain, A., Murphy, E., Nicholl, J.P. (2010). Three techniques for integrating qualitative and quantitative methods in health services research. *BMJ*, **341**, pp. 1147–1150. doi: 10.1136/bmj.c4587.

O'Cathain, A., Thomas, K.J., Drabble, S.J., Rudolph, A., Hewison, J. (2013). What can qualitative research do for randomised controlled trials? A systematic mapping review. *BMJ Open*, **3**(6), p. e002889. doi: 10.1136/bmjopen-2013-002889.

O'Cathain, A., Goode, J., Drabble, S.J., Thomas, K.J., Rudolph, A., Hewison, J. (2014a). Getting added value from using qualitative research with randomised controlled trials: A qualitative interview study. *Trials*, **15**, p. 215. doi: 10.1186/1745-6215-15-215.

O'Cathain, A., Thomas, K.J., Drabble, S.J., Rudolph, A., Goode, J., Hewison, J. (2014b). Maximising the value of combining qualitative research and randomised controlled trials in health research: the QUAlitative Research in Trials (QUART) study—a mixed methods study. *Health Technology Assessment*, **18**(38), pp. 1–197. doi: 10.3310/hta18380.

O'Cathain, A., Hoddinott, P., Lewin, S., Thomas, K.J., Young, B., Adamson, J., Jansen, Y.J.F.M., Mills, N., Moore, G., Donovan, J.L. (2015). Maximising the impact of qualitative research in feasibility studies for randomised controlled trials: guidance for researchers. *Feasibility and Pilot Studies*, **1**, p. 32. doi: 10.1186/s40814-015-0026-y.

O'Cathain, A., Drabble, S.J., Foster, A., Horspool, K., Edwards, L., Thomas, C., Salisbury, C. (2016). Being human: A qualitative interview study exploring why a telehealth intervention for management of chronic conditions had a modest effect. *Journal of Medical Internet Research*, **18**(6), p. e163. doi: 10.2196/jmir.5879.

Parry, G., Power, M. (2016). To RCT or not to RCT? The ongoing saga of randomised trials in quality improvement. *BMJ Qual Saf*, **25**, pp. 221–223. doi:10.1136/bmjqs-2015-004862.

Pawson, R., Tilley, N. (2004). Realist evaluation. In: Matthieson, S. (ed). *Encyclopaedia of evaluation*. Thousand Oaks, CA: Sage Publications.

Penn, C., Evans, M. (2009). Recommendations for communication to enhance informed consent and enrolment at multilingual research sites. *African Journal of AIDS Research*, **8**(3), pp. 285–294. doi: 10.2989/AJAR.2009.8.3.5.926.

Petticrew, M., Rehfuess, E., Noyes, J., Higgins, J., Mayhew, A., Pantoja, T., Shemilt, I., Sowden, A. (2013). Synthesizing evidence on complex interventions: How meta-analytical, qualitative, and mixed-method approaches can contribute. *Journal of Clinical Epidemiology*, **66**(11), pp. 1230–1243. doi: 10.1016/j.jclinepi.2013.06.005.

Petticrew, M., (2015). Time to rethink the systematic review catechism? Moving from 'what works' to 'what happens'. *Systematic Reviews*, **4**, p. 36. doi: 10.1186/s13643-015-0027-1.

Plano Clark V.L., Schumacher, K., West, C., Edrington, J., Dunn, L.B., Harzstark, A., Melisko, M., Rabow, M.W., Swift, P.S., Miaskowski, C. (2013). Practices for embedding an interpretive qualitative approach within a randomized clinical trial. *Journal of Mixed Methods Research*, **7**, pp. 219–242. doi: 10.3310/hta19830.

Popay, J., Williams, G. (1998). Qualitative research and evidence-based healthcare. *Journal of the Royal Society of Medicine*, **91**(35), pp. 32–37.

Pope, C., Mays, N. (1995). Reaching the parts other methods cannot reach: an introduction to qualitative methods in health and health services research. *BMJ*, **311**(6996), pp. 42–45. doi: 10.1136/bmj.311.6996.42.

Pope, C., Mays, N. (eds). (2006). *Qualitative rsearch in health care* (3rd edn). Oxford: Blackwell Publishing (revised edition).

Pope, D.S., Atkins, S., Deluca, A.N., Hausler, H., Hoosain, E., Celentano, D.D., Chaisson, R.E. (2010). South African TB nurses' experiences of provider-initiated HIV counselling and testing in the Eastern Cape Province: A qualitative study. *AIDS Care*, **22**(2), pp. 238–245. doi: 10.1080/09540120903040594.

Prothero, J., Bower, P., Chew-Graham, C. (2007). The use of mixed methodology in evaluating complex interventions: identifying patient factors that moderate the effects of a decision aid. *Family Practice*, **24**, pp. 594–600. doi: 10.1093/fampra/cmm066.

Punch, K.F. (2016). *Developing effective research proposals* (3rd edn). Thousand Oaks, CA: Sage Publications.

Raine, R., Fitzpatrick, R., Barratt, H., Bevan, G., Black, N., Boaden, R., Bower, P., Campbell, M., Denis, J.L., Devers, K., Dixon-Woods, M., Fallowfield, L., Forder, J., Foy, R., Freemantle, N., Fulop, N.J., Gibbons, E., Gillies, C., Goulding, L., Grieve, R., Grimshaw, J., Howarth, E., Lilford, R.J., McDonald, R., Moore, G., Moore, L., Newhouse, R., O'Cathain, A., Or, Z., Papoutsi, C., Prady, S., Rycroft-Malone, J., Sekhon, J., Turner, S., Watson, S.I., Zwarenstein, M. (2016). Challenges, solutions and future directions in the evaluation of service innovations in health care and public health. *Health Services and Delivery Research*, **4**, p. 16.

Rapport, F., Storey, M., Porter, A., Snooks, H., Jones, K., Peconi, J., Sánchez, A., Siebert, S., Thorne, K., Clement, C., Russell, I. (2013). Qualitative research within trials: developing a standard operating procedure for a Clinical Trials Unit. *Trials*, **14**, p. 54. doi: 10.1186/1745-6215-14-54.

Riley, T., Hawe, P., Shiell, A. (2005). Contested ground: How should qualitative evidence inform the conduct of a community intervention trial? *Journal of Health Services Research & Policy*, **10**(2), pp. 103–110. doi: 10.1258/1355819053559029.

Ritchie, J., Spencer, L. (1994). Qualitative data analysis for applied policy research. In: Bryman, A., Burgess, R. (eds). *Analysing qualitative data*. London: Routledge, pp. 173–194.

Ritchie, J., Lewis, J. (2013). *Qualitative research practice: a guide for social science students and researchers* (2nd edn). Thousand Oaks, CA: Sage Publications.

Romo, N., Poo, M., and **Ballesta, R.** (2009). From illegal poison to legal medicine: A qualitative research in a heroin-prescription trial in Spain. *Drug and alcohol review*, **28**(2), pp. 186–195. doi: 10.1111/j.1465-3362.2008.00015.x.

Rooshenas, L., Mcmullen, C., Mathers, J., Townsend, D., Donovan, J., Blazeby, J. (2015). How pre-trial qualitative research can change proposed RCT design: a case study and implications for future research. *Trials*, **16**(Suppl. 2), p. O35. doi: 10.1186/1745-6215-16-S2-O35.

Salisbury, C., O'Cathain, A., Edwards, L., Thomas, C., Gaunt, D., Hollinghurst, S., Nicholl, J., Large, S., Yardley, L., Lewis, G., Foster, A., Garner, K., Horspool, K., Man, M.S., Rogers, A., Pope, C., Dixon, P., Montgomery, A.A. (2016). Effectiveness of an integrated telehealth service for patients with depression: a pragmatic randomised controlled trial of a complex intervention. *Lancet, Psychiatry*, **3**(6), pp. 515–525. doi: 10.1016/S2215-0366(16)00083-3.

Salisbury, C., O'Cathain, A., Thomas, C., Edwards, L., Montgomery, A.A., Hollinghurst, S., Large, S., Nicholl, J., Pope, C., Rogers, A., Lewis, G., Fahey, T., Yardley, L.,

Brownsell, S., Dixon, P., Drabble, S., Esmonde, L., Foster, A., Garner, K., Gaunt, D., Horspool, K., Man, M., Rowsell, A., Segar, J. (2017). An evidence-based approach to the use of telehealth in long-term health conditions: development of an intervention and evaluation through pragmatic randomised controlled trials in patients with depression or raised cardiovascular risk. *Programme Grants for Applied Research*, **5**, p. 1. doi: 10.3310/pgfar05010.

Sandelowski, M, (1996). Using qualitative methods in intervention studies. *Research in Nursing & Health*, **19**, pp. 359–364. doi: 10.1002/(SICI)1098-240X(199608)19:4<359::AID-NUR9>3.0.CO;2-H.

Sandelowski, M., and **Barroso, J.** (2003). Writing the proposal for a qualitative research methodology project. *Qualitative Health Research*, **13**(6), pp. 781–820.doi: 10.1177/1049732303013006003.

Sawtell, M., Jamieson, L., Wiggins, M., Smith, F., Ingold, A., Hargreaves, K., Khatwa, M., Brooks, L., Thompson, R., Christie, D. (2015). Implementing a structured education program for children with diabetes: Lessons learnt from an integrated process evaluation. *BMJ Open Diabetes Research & Care*, **3**(1), e000065. doi: 10.1136/bmjdrc-2014-000065.

Schumacher, K.L., Koresawa, S., West, C., Dodd, M., Paul, S.M., Tripathy, P., Koo, P., Miaskowski, C. (2005). Qualitative research contribution to a randomized clinical trial. *Research in Nursing and Health*, **28**(3), pp. 268–280. doi: 10.1002/nur.20080.

SCT (2013) 34th Annual Meeting, Boston, Massachusetts, USA, May 19–22, http://www.sctweb.org/public/meetings/2013/home.cfm

Shagi, C., Vallely, A., Kasindi, S., Chiduo, B., Desmond, N., Soteli, S., Kavit, N., Vallely, L., Lees, S., Hayes, R., Ross, D. (2008). A model for community representation and participation in HIV prevention trials among women who engage in transactional sex in Africa. *AIDS Care*, **20**(9), pp. 1039–1049. doi: 10.1080/09540120701842803.

Silverman, S.L. (2013). *Doing qualitative research*. Thousand Oaks, CA: Sage Publications.

Simons, L. (2007). Moving from collision to integration. Reflecting on the experience of mixed methods. *Journal of Research in Nursing*, **12**, pp. 73–83. doi:10.1177/1744987106069514.

Smith, J. A., Flowers, P., Larkin, M. (2009). *Interpretative phenomenological analysis: theory, method and research*. London: Sage Publications.

Smith, J.D., Baillie, J., Baglin, T., O'Griffiths, G., Casbard, A., Cohen D., Fitzmaurice, D.A., Hood, K., Rose, P., Cohen, A.T., Johnson, M., Maraveyas, A., Bell, J., Toone, H., Nelson, A., Noble, S.I. (2014). A feasibility study to inform the design of a randomized controlled trial to identify the most clinically and cost effective Anticoagulation Length with low molecular weight heparin in the treatment of Cancer Associated Thrombosis (ALICAT): study protocol for a mixed-methods study. *Trials*, **15**, 122. doi: 10.1186/1745-6215-15-122.

Sniehotta, F., Presseau, J., Hobbs, N., Araújo-Soares, V. (2012). Testing self-regulation interventions to increase walking using factorial randomized N-of-1 trials. *Health Psychology*, **31**(6), pp. 733–737. doi: 10.1037/a0027337.

Snowdon, C., Brocklehurst, P., Tasker, R., Ward Platt, M., Harvey, S., Elbourne, D. (2014). Death, bereavement and randomised controlled trials (BRACELET): a methodological study of policy and practice in neonatal and paediatric intensive care trials. *Health Technology Assessment*, **18**(42), pp. 1–410. doi: 10.3310/hta18420.

Song, M.K., Ward, S.E., Happ, M.B., Piraino, B., Donovan, H.S., Shields, A.M., Connolly, M.C. (2009). Randomized controlled trial of SPIRIT: an effective approach to preparing African-American dialysis patients and families for end of life. *Research in Nursing & Health*, **32**(3), pp. 260–273, doi: 10.1002/nur.20320.

Song, M.K., Sandelowski, M., Happ, M.B. (2010). Current practices and emerging trends in conducting mixed methods intervention studies in health sciences. In Tashakkori A., and Teddlie C. (eds), *Mixed methods in social & behavioural research* (2nd edn). Thousand Oaks, CA: Sage Publications, pp. 725–747.

Stapleton, H., Kirkham, M., Thomas G. (2002). Qualitative study of evidence based leaflets in maternity care. *BMJ (Clinical research ed.)*, **324**(7338), p. 639. doi: 10.1136/bmj.324.7338.639.

Strauss, A., Corbin, J. (1990). *Basics of qualitative research: grounded theory*. Thousand Oaks, CA: Sage Publications.

Teddlie, C., Tashakkori, A. (2008). *foundations of mixed methods research: integrating quantitative and qualitative approaches in the social and behavioral sciences*. Thousand Oaks, CA: Sage Publications.

Thomas, C., Man, M.S., O'Cathain, A., Hollinghurst, S., Large, S., Edwards, L., Nicholl, J., Montgomery, A., Salisbury, C. (2014). Effectiveness and cost-effectiveness of a telehealth intervention to support the management of long-term conditions: study protocol for two linked randomized controlled trials. *Trials*, **15**, 36. doi: 10.1186/1745-6215-15-36.

Thorne, S. (2008). *Interpretive description*. Walnut Creek, CA: Left Coast Press.

Thorstensson, C.A., Lohmander, L.S., Frobell, R.B., Roos, E.M., Gooberman-Hill, R. (2009). Choosing surgery: patients' preferences within a trial of treatments for anterior cruciate ligament injury. A qualitative study. *BMC Musculoskeletal Disorders*, **10**, p. 100. doi: 10.1186/1471-2474-10-100.

Tong, A., Sainsbury, P., Craig, J. (2007). Consolidated criteria for reporting qualitative research (COREQ): a 32-item checklist for interviews and focus groups. *International Journal for Quality in Healthcare*, **19**(6), pp. 349–357. doi: 10.1093/intqhc/mzm042.

Tonkin-Crine, S., Anthierens, S., Francis, N.A., Brugman, C., Fernandez-Vandellos, P., Krawczyk, J., Llor, C., Yardley, L., Coenen, S., Godycki-Cwirko, M., Butler, C.C., Verheij, T.J., Goossens, H., Little, P., Cals, J.W., GRACE INTRO team. (2014). Exploring patients' views of primary care consultations with contrasting interventions for acute cough: a six-country European qualitative study. *Primary Care Respiratory Medicine*, **24**, p. 14026. doi: 10.1038/npjpcrm.2014.26.

Tonkin-Crine, S., Anthierens, S., Hood, K., Yardley, L., Cals, J.W.L., Francis, N.A., Coenen, S., van der Velden, A.W., Godycki-Cwirko, M., Llor, C., Butler, C.C., Verheij, T.J.M., Goossens, H., Little, P., on behalf of the GRACE INTRO/CHAMP consortium. (2016). Discrepancies between qualitative and quantitative evaluation of randomised controlled trial results: Achieving clarity through mixed methods triangulation. *Implementation Science*, **11**, p. 66. doi: 10.1186/s13012-016-0436-0.

Torgerson, D.J., Torgerson, C. J. (2008). *Designing randomised trials in health, education and the social sciences: an introduction*. Basingstoke: Palgrave Macmillan.

Toye, F., Williamson, E., Williams, M.A., Fairbank, J., Lamb, S.E. (2016). What value can qualitative research add to quantitative research design? An example from an adolescent idiopathic scoliosis trial feasibility study. *Qualitative Health Research*, pp. 1–13(s). doi: 10.1177/1049732316662446.

Treweek, S., Zwarenstein, M. (2009). Making trials matter: pragmatic and explanatory trials and the problem of applicability. *Trials*, **10**, 37. doi: 10.1186/1745-6215-10-37.

Trickett, E.J. (2011). Community-based participatory research as worldview or instrumental strategy: is it lost in translation(al) research? *American Journal of Public Health*, **101**(8), pp. 1353–1355. doi: 10.2105/AJPH.2011.300124.

Van Ness, P.H., Murphy, T.E., Ather, A. (2016). Attention to individuals: mixed methods for N-of-1 health care interventions. *Journal of Mixed Methods Research*, **11**(3), pp. 342–354. doi: 10.1177/1558689815623685.

Waheed, W., Hughes-Morley, A., Woodham, A., Allen, G., Bower, P. (2015). Overcoming barriers to recruiting ethnic minorities to mental health research: a typology of recruitment strategies. *BMC Psychiatry*, **15**, p. 101. doi:10.1186/s12888-015-0484-z.

Walley, J.D., Khan, M.A., Newell, J.N., Khan, M.H. (2001). Effectiveness of the direct observation component of DOTS for tuberculosis: a randomised controlled trial in Pakistan. *Lancet*, **357**(9257), pp. 664–669. doi: 10.1016/S0140-6736(00)04129-5.

Wells, M., Williams, B., Treweek, S., Coyle, J., Taylor, J. (2012). Intervention description is not enough: evidence from an in-depth multiple case study on the untold role and impact of context in randomised controlled trials of seven complex interventions. *Trials*, **13**(1), p. 95. doi: 10.1186/1745-6215-13-95.

White, E., Winstanley, J. (2009). Implementation of clinical supervision: educational preparation and subsequent diary accounts of the practicalities involved, from an Australian mental health [corrected] nursing innovation. *Journal of Psychiatric and Mental Health Nursing*, **16**, pp. 895–903. doi: 10.1111/j.1365-2850.2009.01466.x.

Wiart, L., Rosychuk, R.J., Wright, F.V. (2016). Evaluation of the effectiveness of robotic gait training and gait-focused physical therapy programs for children and youth with cerebral palsy: a mixed methods RCT. *BMC Neurology*, **16**, 86. doi: 10.1186/s12883-016-0582-7.

Yin, R.K. (2003). *Case study research: design and methods: applied social research methods* (5th edn). Thousand Oaks, CA: Sage Publications.

Index

Tables and boxes are indicated by an italic *t* or *b* following the page number.

Made in the USA
Monee, IL
13 September 2026

62978026R00122